I0096818

Skin Care

Ancient Indian Remedies for Skin Conditions

(Complete Guide to Korean Beauty Using Natural Ingredients)

Danny Gonzalez

Published By **Phil Dawson**

Danny Gonzalez

Skin Care: Ancient Indian Remedies for Skin Conditions (Complete Guide to Korean Beauty Using Natural Ingredients)

ISBN   978-1-998038-76-3

No part of this guidebook shall be reproduced in any form without permission in writing from the publisher except in the case of brief quotations embodied in critical articles or reviews.

Legal & Disclaimer

The information contained in this book is not designed to replace or take the place of any form of medicine or professional medical advice. The information in this book has been provided for educational & entertainment purposes only.

The information contained in this book has been compiled from sources deemed reliable, and it is accurate to the best of the Author's knowledge; however, the Author cannot guarantee its accuracy and validity and cannot be held liable for any errors or omissions. Changes are periodically made to this book. You must consult your doctor or get professional medical advice before using any of the suggested remedies, techniques, or information in this book.

Table Of Contents

Chapter 1: What is a great morning skin care ordinary?

This will depend on a couple of factors: how lots time you want/have available to spend and your pores and pores and skin kind.

A number one ordinary ought to in all likelihood look like this:

Cleanse

Tone

Treat

Eye/Lip

SPF/Moisturizer

If you are any man or woman who's a definitely oily pores and pores and skin type - and through the use of that, I suggest that you awaken inside the morning with form of a waxy buildup for your pores and skin - you may want initially cleanse, then examine the final steps for your liking/time.

If you're every body who has extra ordinary/mixture or dry/sensitive pores and skin, you could pick out to bypass a cleanse inside the morning and pass right now to toner. What? Did I just blow your thoughts? If you are washing your sheets and towels regularly, you will be a tremendous candidate to pass a cleanse proper proper right here and there. However, do not do this if you are not washing towels/sheets frequently as you will need to clean that buildup off.

Treat is probably something like a nutrition C serum, hyaluronic acid, a few aspect that has a flash tightening impact.

If you are not a dry pores and skin type or do not stay in a completely dry climate, you may possibly pass moisturizer and simply use SPF to your morning regular.

What is a first rate night time time skin care routine?

Evening is the right time to deep clean your skin, thereby casting off the environmental pollution (pollutants), buildup, make-up residue, and bacteria at the pores and pores and skin earlier than smooshing your face on a pillow for numerous hours. Sounds like a excellent concept, right?

The ordinary appears similar to the morning ordinary:

Cleanse

Tone

Treat

Eye/Lip

Moisturize

Everyone, and I do recommend every body, have to cleanse at night. Follow with a toner to repair the proper pH stability, then cope with. Treat at night time time should consist of factors like an exfoliation serum, acne remedy, or retinol. They also can include your morning remedies, however the ones I've indexed here are most effective at night time

time time at the identical time as you relaxation.

The special exchange is plain;, you do not want an SPF at the same time as you sleep, so just use the right moisturizer to your skin.

Is having one sort of pores and skin better or worse than every other?

There is not any "horrible" pores and pores and skin; it does no longer choose out to "misbehave." However, pores and skin may be complicated. It modifications each day based mostly on many different factors we disclose it to, like food, water, operating out, weather, pollutants, how we take care of it, show screen time, and extra.

Learning the way to deal with extremely good complications is exactly why you picked up this e-book, proper?!

What is one component I can do for higher skin in recent times?

The extraordinary things you can do in your pores and pores and skin to make terrific trade *nearly* proper now and prolonged-time period:

☐ hydrat

☐ consume more culmination and veggies

☐ placed on sunscreen every day– sure, even inside the wintry weather, even indoors

☐ decide to a skincare recurring that works in your pores and pores and skin

SPF – What, When, Where, How, and Why??

What to Apply:

Using no longer much less than SPF 30 each day will ensure you take specific care of your skin and assisting to prevent signs and signs and symptoms of having vintage and pores and skin most cancers.

When to Apply:

Fifteen mins earlier than going outside, and reapply every hours.

Where to Apply:

Anywhere there may be pores and skin! Except your eyelids.

But in all seriousness, some of the most typically left out areas are our hairline, the element in our hair, our ears, the backs of our arms, and the tops of our ft. Don't bypass these regions!

How Much to Apply:

An ounce should be sufficient to cowl maximum humans each two hours. Think of the dimensions of a mean shot glass, it truly is an oz... Now thinking to your self "sh*t...I in reality don't use that a bargain?" properly now you apprehend better, so that you can do higher, right?

Another manner to think about this? Look at how many oz.. Are to your bottle of sunscreen...The common is 8 oz. That have to be eight packages each hours. So in case you're outdoor for eight hours inside the destiny, because of this half of of your bottle of sunscreen need to be long long past.

Set an alarm in your watch or phone for every hours you may be outside.

Why This Is So Important:

There isn't always any man or woman product extra important in preventing pores and pores and skin most cancers and signs of growing older than your SPF. Find ones you like and do not forget to inventory up.

I'm on a budget - what are the most vital products to spend money on?

When using Professional Grade products, normally you want to apply plenty tons a great deal much less of the product than maximum drugstore and branch shop products. This manner you may each store cash or spend the same quantity long term, at the same time as getting better top notch materials that might create real trade within the pores and skin. For instance, your cleaner may want to possibly very last a month or with a much less highly-priced one (AKA mass marketplace) costs $10, however in case you spend $35 at the most effective from your esthetician, it's miles probable to last 4-6 months whilst used effectively.

If you need to pick out, I need to endorse spending your coins on topics that stay for your face - toners, remedies, eye cream, and moisturizers. Save your cash on matters similar to the purifier and make-up remover you wash off.

Professional Products

Mass Market Products

☐ Small batches

☐ Large batches

☐ More energetic factors

☐ Less energetic elements

☐ Stronger method

☐

Weaker method

☐ Higher extremely good additives

☐ Lower excellent additives

☐ Delivery structures which allow for better penetration of energetic additives

☐ Delivery systems which don't allow for correct penetration of lively substances

☐ Concentrated formulas

☐ Not targeted system

Chapter 2: What is the exquisite order to use my skincare products?

The fashionable rule is to apply so as through using the use of weight:

1.Cleanser

2.Toner

3.Serum

four.Eye Cream

5.Moisturizer

6.Oil

7.SPF

Obviously, you can pass over some of the ones steps primarily based honestly at the day, time of day, or honestly because you do not use it. Just skip that step and flow into to the subsequent item you do use.

Can I use products from multiple manufacturers?

Absolutely, you could! As someone who has advanced a skin care line, I would love for everybody to be the usage of all of my stuff. However, I in fact apprehend that there is probably a product from a few different line that they truely love and they may see the effects they want from it. I moreover recognize there are positive things missing from my line, like benzoyl peroxide merchandise. Until I can carry those missing components to the desk, I cannot sincerely say that I in fact have the whole thing for all people, so I do inspire humans to look some distinct place for the things that I do now not have.

However, even as you are blending strains, you want to make sure you aren't overdoing exfoliating. For instance, if your serum has retinol from one line, and your night time time cream has it from every other line, you're doing double responsibility and that could worsen your pores and pores and skin.

In skin care, it's far extra approximately what is strolling for you in place of what line it comes from.

I recognize this isn't a well-known opinion – however I've in no manner been one to inform you what's famous, I'm the friend who will inform you the truth.

Do I really need an afternoon cream and a night time time time cream?

Whether or no longer you'll use the same moisturizer at night time in preference to day depends at the factors. You sincerely should trade it up primarily based at the truth which you need to use an SPF at some stage in the day and no SPF at night time time.

However, if you are a person who has dry pores and pores and skin and goals the extra moisturizer in the end of the day, you could choose to layer your moisturizer under your SPF and use that identical moisturizer at night time time time too, if it's miles not an exfoliating (i.E., solar sensitizing) moisturizer.

Do I really need an eye constant cream?

The short answer is positive, I could suggest an eye cream to each person, any age. The pores and skin round our eyes is the thinnest on our frame - about the thickness of tissue paper - and therefore needs particularly formulated merchandise a good way to no longer clog the pores within the area and will accommodate the sensitive nature of the pores and pores and skin there.

While we are proper proper here, permit's communicate approximately how to comply with eye cream properly. Using your ring finger, tap a tiny amount round your orbital bone. Don't placed eye cream any inside the direction of the attention than that, because it will migrate into your eye simply from the natural moves of your eyes, even in your sleep. You can lightly massage the attention cream in, being careful now not to stretch or pull the pores and skin spherical the eye, and transferring outward in the direction of your temple for exquisite de-puffing effects.

How lengthy is my product accurate for?

Most merchandise are shelf-sturdy for one to 3 years in their jar unopened. Oftentimes, products have a touch jar photo within the back of the package cope with the aim to have a touch range (like six, twelve, twenty-4, and so on.) in it so it seems like a touch rectangle with a flip pinnacle. That's how long the product is proper for as quickly as you have got opened it in months. That being said, it does no longer imply that the product itself right now may be awful at that month mark. It way that it becomes a good buy less powerful, and may start harboring bacteria. However, I could enjoy assured the use of it for a few more weeks if the following conditions are met: it appears, smells, and feels similar to it did while you opened it. If any of these topics have changed, I may toss it and cope with your self to a modern-day one.

When have to I see a dermatologist in region of an esthetician?

My recommendation is that everybody sees their dermatologist as quick as a 12 months for an basic frame test of their skin, moles, for a pores and skin maximum cancers test, and every time they've got a subject about any sort of pores and pores and skin infections that would require medication.

I endorse seeing an esthetician for nearly all fantastic pores and pores and skin issues. We are educated to have a look at the general health of the skin, your way of life, and plenty of particular factors to expand a remedy plan and regular a great manner to be honestly right for you. We generally have extra time set aside to train you about your pores and pores and skin and why you will want to use a specific trouble or prevent doing or the usage of one.

Can pores and skin acclimate to a product so it stops running? I've heard I must alternate topics up so my skin doesn't "get used to" a product…

No, now not in reality, but furthermore sure.

If you start using a current product and also you experience any redness or contamination right away, however then your pores and skin calms all of the manner proper right down to it after some makes use of, your pores and pores and skin has acclimated to the product. A correct example of this will be retinol or glycolic acid.

Your pores and skin has technically acclimated to a product, however that doesn't propose it stopped strolling. It manner that it's miles adjusted to what changed into previously demanding that cellular turnover.

If we are talking approximately things like a cleanser or a toner, no your pores and skin may want to not get acclimated. If it stops strolling as well because it once did for you, in all likelihood both the product has expired or your pores and skin has modified and it's time to visit a expert to get a more up to date normal installation for you.

What is a double cleanse? Do I need to try this?

Double cleaning is the use of a pre-purifier like a facial oil or micellar water to break down the makeup it's far for your pores and pores and pores and skin in order that your cleanser can wash the whole lot away.

The steps to a double cleanse:

1) Use your oil or micellar water on the pores and pores and skin.

a) If the use of oil, practice a few drops and massage over pores and pores and skin, then gently wipe away residue in advance than moving right now to Step 2.

b) If using micellar water, you follow that to a cotton round or towel and wipe over pores and pores and skin gently, then drift at once to Step 2.

2) Cleanse as regular, following up with the relaxation of your ordinary.

Double cleaning isn't a crucial step for everyone. Here's a short check you may do at domestic to determine if you want to be:

• First, are you cleaning for ninety seconds? If not, begin there.

• After you cleanse for ninety seconds, use a toner on a cotton spherical or white towel. Is there any color deposited onto the cotton spherical or white towel? If so, you want to double cleanse.

How prolonged will or no longer it's miles till I see effects from a current day product I'm using?

That really is based upon on plenty of factors. As adults, our pores and skin cells shed (AKA turn over) shape of each 30 days, so you'll typically have the ability to inform if a product is really working for you at approximately a month. However, if it's far a top notch expert product, you may see outcomes interior days.

If you are trying a brand new product, deliver it a few weeks to look exchange besides it's inflicting an hypersensitive reaction or an excessive amount of sensitivity.

Do I need a mini refrigerator for my pores and skin care?

No, you do not need one; it's miles a preference. I use mine to keep my sheet masks and my eye cream bloodless further to my face curler and my gua sha stones.

I really like having access to the less warm gear and lotions inside the morning to help reduce puffiness. It's fresh and soothing and strikes a chord in my memory that I'm doing some factor for myself.

Can't I absolutely use my body lotion on my face?

No, you can not. Sorry for my bluntness there, however this has to stop ASAP. Body creams are formulated for the thicker pores and pores and skin it is on our our our bodies and typically has extra quantities of comedogenic elements in it.

Professional pores and pores and skin care formulated in your face has the right pH balance to get the factors where they want to go to create trade in the pores and skin, is non-comedogenic, and is formulated for the thinner facial skin.

Chapter 3: How do I cast off darkish circles?

Unfortunately, darkish circles are each hereditary, because of dietary factors, sleep deprivation, developing vintage, alcohol consumption, or allergic reactions. There isn't honestly an eye fixed fixed cream to be able to certainly eliminate them. In an eye fixed steady cream, caffeine and food plan K can assist lower the advent of darkish circles, and an tremendous concealer works wonders.

How can I deliver all of my pores and pores and skin care with me as soon as I journey?

I propose that my clients spend money on a adventure set in their preferred merchandise after which fill up those bottles from their massive set simply so they may be now not contributing to landfill waste.

Another couple of options in case you choose:

get a hard and speedy of adventure bottles from the shop and fill those. Just make certain you label them and both placed tape over the marker, or use an real label maker, simply so they labels are water resistant.

-OR-

Pick up multiple touch lens instances, and top off those.

Why is exfoliation critical?

When you have a take a look at a pass-section of pores and pores and skin underneath a immoderate powered microscope, it looks as if layers of bricks on pinnacle of every precise. (Yes, it's miles an great over-simplification, however go through with me.) When you accept as true with you studied of a brick pattern, staggered bricks, with the cement in amongst them to hold them collectively, it's a notable analogy of the manner the cells line up first of all.

Now accept as true with our "brick wall" however at the lowest of the wall are plump, juicy grapes. Those are our "infant" pores and pores and skin cells. As they go with the flow up toward the floor, they flatten out and emerge as extra like raisins.

So a lot of how we deal with our pores and pores and skin is based on facts that simple concept, so look at it again until you get it, ok? I promise it's far going to be virtually really worth it.

Exfoliation is critical because of the truth our pores and pores and skin is in particular proper at protecting itself. The "intracellular cement" that holds the dried and shriveled up "raisin" cells at the pinnacle layer is difficult. So we cut up the bonds maintaining that collectively, and go along with the flow those "raisin" cells away, leaving the extra plump and juicy searching "grape" cells seen.

Also, whilst those "raisin" cells are sitting on top of the pores and pores and skin, they prevent a number of the lively components for your pores and skin care from getting in which they want to visit make modifications inside the pores and pores and pores and skin. So exfoliating in truth makes your specific products art work higher.

You do now not want to over-exfoliate even though both. If you do, your pores and pores and skin can emerge as sensitive, overly dry, crimson or itchy, and reactive. So sure, exfoliate. Regularly. But don't overdo it both.

What kind of excfoliant is exceptional for my pores and pores and skin kind?

There are two forms of exfoliants: chemical and bodily (additionally referred to as manual). Chemical exfoliants are things like enzymes, lactic acid peels, retinol, and plenty of greater. These artwork by using way of dissolving the bonds that keep skin cells together.

A guide exfoliant is something that scrubs like a rice scrub, walnut scrub, or perhaps dermaplaning or microdermabrasion. These paintings thru manually breaking aside the vain pores and skin cells and sloughing them away.

My belief is that every sorts can be proper for all and sundry. For instance, I recommend a retinol serum, a glycolic acid toner, and a rice polish to a variety of my clients. It's all about spacing matters out and ensuring your pores and pores and skin can tolerate it.

A properly large exfoliation plan might also additionally want to appearance some aspect like this (in case you are the usage of retinol 2x in step with week)

Sunday night time time: retinol

Monday night time: glycolic toner

Tuesday night time: wreck

Wednesday morning: polish

Thursday night: retinol

Friday night time: glycolic toner

Saturday morning: polish

This ordinary would not paintings for all and sundry, however it's an instance of a way to spread out exfoliants so you do no longer overdo it, but however get the advantage of every type.

Is it ok to DIY my skincare or make my private at-domestic masks?

I do now not endorse it. I'll admit as soon as I turn out to be a youngster, I did mess around with some of that stuff (it is a chunk little little bit of foreshadowing for me looking to create a pores and skin care line as an person). However, there are a few certainly crucial reasons why I could no longer want you to DIY skin care now that I realize extra about formulations.

First, you do not know how active an detail can be. For instance, pineapple is an factor that is utilized in pretty some professional exfoliants. However, the ones are less probably to motive any issues like chemical burns or hypersensitive reactions because they may be pH balanced properly for the meant use and pores and pores and skin reputation. Unless you check it, how do you apprehend the pH of the pineapple you're using?

We additionally do no longer realize what type of microbes is probably in there in case you honestly pop a pineapple in a blender and slap a layer for your skin.

If you'll do it in any case (due to the fact I apprehend a number of your will, le sigh), right right right here are my suggestions to lower your chance of burns and infections:

1) Sterilize the whole thing that you're going to apply earlier.

2) Pick only one element to use if you do have a reaction, so you realise what it changed into you reacted to.

3) Don't maintain it; throw away any leftover right now

4) Don't use pure vital oils right away at the pores and skin; they will be too strong for that. You need to dilute them with a few issue and constantly do a patch check first.

Does my healthy eating plan in reality have an impact on my pores and skin?

Absolutely it could and it does! Every day our pores and pores and skin modifications based on what we've got got had to devour, drink, what medicines and vitamins we have taken, and so forth. It changes primarily based on our surroundings round us, much like the weather, whether or not or not we are in a dry or humid room, indoor heating, and so on.

The lesson right here is to consume as many stop end result and veggies as you may, in a large shape of shades. Eat wholesome fat, drink water, and cope with your self. Your pores and pores and skin shows the way you deal with your self. If you really eat junk, you're treating your pores and pores and skin like junk.

Chapter 4: How lots water need to I in fact be ingesting?

That's a definitely proper question and it varies with the useful useful resource of person. The antique adage of six to eight glasses an afternoon isn't always actual anymore. It definitely is primarily based upon on our manner of lifestyles, any drug treatments we're taking, what we devour, how a lot we exercising, and our fashionable surroundings. If you live in a dry weather you could not understand which you're sweating because the sweat evaporates off of you straight away.

A standard variety for most people is to drink 1/2 of of your frame weight in ozin step with day. For example, if you weigh a hundred and fifty kilos, you need to motive for seventy five ozof water every day. Be sure to update fluids misplaced while exercise, heavy sweating, or have been ill.

Something else to phrase, culmination and vegetable intake counts within the course of your water intake as properly. Eating loads of produce has pores and pores and skin advantages that drift an extended manner past the water they contain, so consume masses of them, and a massive form of them!

Remember, if you are thirsty, you are already dehydrated, but mild it is able to be.

If your lips are dry, you are already dehydrated.

If your urine is yellow to dark yellow, you are already dehydrated.

If you are experiencing fatigue or dizziness, you're already dehydrated.

If you need to transport deep into the research, you can go to the ones net web web page or look at this e-book as properly!

Book: Quench with the aid of the usage of Dana Cohen, M.D. And Gina Bria

Does drinking from a straw purpose wrinkles?

Sadly, sure, and alas, the ones are a number of the maximum difficult and painful wrinkles to deal with. If you consider anybody who modified proper right into a smoker, they nearly all have wrinkles spherical their mouth.

The equal movement to puff on a cigarette is crucial to drink from a straw. Unfortunately, I'm one of these people that liquids extra water if I'm ingesting out of a cup with a straw, so I'm on foot on lowering that dependancy going ahead. However, I'm moreover normally weighing the venture of being hydrated as opposed to wrinkles, and hydrated wins, so choose out out your poison.

When want to I start the use of anti-growing older merchandise?

Let's begin with the resource of clarifying what we are regarding as anti-growing older for the sake of this question and solution. I'm regarding retinol, brightening products like vitamins C and Kojic acid, SPF, and pores and pores and skin toning peptides on the same time as talking approximately anti-growing older products.

Starting to apply them in your overdue young adults, early twenties will help prevent a few signs and signs of getting vintage, so the sooner you operate them, the higher. In truth, my primary recommendation for anti-developing older is sporting SPF each day, as young as viable, together with toddlers, babies, and so on.

To be flawlessly clean, this does not endorse that in case you are for your thirties, forties, or perhaps seventies and eighties which you could not see consequences. Any age can see outcomes with additives aimed in the direction of lowering signs of getting antique. It's the distinction between prevention and reduction of gift signs and symptoms and symptoms and signs.

How can I avoid wrinkles?

There are such plenty of factors that may purpose wrinkles, I cannot list the entirety proper right here, but I can provide you with some elegant hints that I would possibly inform everyone:

1.Always, typically, continuously placed on sunscreen. This should not need elaboration proper now, with all the information we've now, however for the sake of this e book....Here ya skip: SPF is the only thing we recognize for terrific can help save you symptoms and signs and symptoms of having old. WEAR IT.

2.Build a strong habitual and be committed to that routine, adjusting as needed - seasonally, day by day, with age. That approach seeing a expert to help you choose the right merchandise to your skin and making the modifications which might be critical to preserve your pores and pores and skin inside the remarkable state of affairs it could be through the years.

3.Use retinol. It allows construct collagen, reduces breakouts, reduces hyperpigmentation. It's basically an all-round product that nearly everyone can advantage from. But, you want to place on sunscreen while using it, as your pores and pores and pores and skin is more likely to burn.

4.Be aware of the expressions you're making. Obviously, I'm no longer going to tell you to prevent smiling. But have in thoughts of things like while you're looking your computer screen, are you frowning? Furrowing your brow? Attempt to loosen up those muscles while you may.

five.Manage your strain degrees as remarkable as you may. Cortisol breaks down collagen, the plumping a part of the pores and skin. Have you ever seen a time-lapse photo of a U.S. President on the start in their time period in choice to the cease? The big difference in their face over four to eight years is exquisite, and is probable because of elements of the continual stress prompted through the use of the use of their manner.

Authors Note: Dear President Obama,

I suggest no disrespect, and please forgive

me using you for example.

I preference you may see that it changed into intended

for educational features.

Do I need to alter my skincare seasonally?

Some human beings don't want to, however others do, in particular if you stay in a completely humid or very bloodless surroundings. If you stay in a extra moderate temperature region, you may or may not want to.

Here's an example of why you would in all likelihood need to adjust your normal seasonally:

If you stay in an area like I do (shout out Minnesota!), within the wintry climate, it may get into the bad 60s for the temperature outside. But, while we come interior to a heated environment, it is sixty five-seventy five stages. That's greater or an awful lot much less a a hundred-degree swing in seconds. Obviously, it isn't constantly like that, but it isn't always extraordinarily uncommon both. Even a swing of 32 ranges out of doors to 70 levels internal is enough to throw off your skin's moisture barrier.

If you stay in a extraordinary humid weather (shout out south Florida!), you'll be dealing with some factor like humid out of doors, dry indoors, and overheating at the same time as outdoor.

Should I change my pores and skin care primarily based on the seasons? Weather? My age?

The solution is sure, to all of those topics. I recommend maximum human beings have some merchandise in their pores and pores and skin care arsenal with the intention to deal with particular seasons or temperatures and the way their pores and skin is responding at any given time.

I additionally advise that people paintings with an esthetician frequently as a manner to hold to prevent signs and symptoms and symptoms of developing older, alter to cutting-edge way of life changes or body changes, and deal with signs and symptoms of having older as they mature as nicely.

Can I surely prevent stretchmarks?

Yes, and no. You can lessen your opportunities of getting stretch marks with the beneficial resource of retaining your pores and skin hydrated externally and internally, and consuming correct nutritious food.

At a few issue in our lives, but, maximum people do growth stretch marks, so don't beat your self up over them. Some of this is genetic, a number of it's miles environmental and because of fluctuations in weight. I bear in thoughts analyzing about a person calling her stretch marks from being pregnant "tiger stripes" and I genuinely cherished that concept; mamas are tigers for nice.

The specific information is, most stretch marks start out shape of purple searching and grow to be extra flesh-toned over the path of time, therefore turning into much less noticeabl

Why doesn't this product that everybody loves paintings for me?

Everyone's skin is distinct. Just because your bestie or mom or all of us else loves it would not suggest that your pores and skin loves it. Using a one-of-a-type instance, there are certain colorings that appearance first rate on my sister but don't look particular on me honestly due to a mild distinction in our pores and pores and skin tone or our hair colour. Now think about that on a cellular diploma and the manner your cells are in truth not prepared to handle that specific product and feature it create notable alternate in your pores and skin.

So to take it with a grain of salt and speak over with a expert who will let you simply slim down what the right components for your pores and pores and skin are to accumulate the effects you're looking for.

Chapter 5: Why should I use a satin or silk pillowcase?

It permits prevent friction and could growth slip on the pores and skin, which decreases wrinkles and wonderful traces. It furthermore prevents the horrifying crease mark from a pillowcase whilst you awaken after an amazing prolonged sleep. It may not help with breakouts despite the fact that, so I notwithstanding the reality that advise that you exchange your pillowcase as a minimum as speedy as in line with week.

If you are a person who likes their pillows to in shape, I advocate getting a satin or silk pillowcase for each pillow of the mattress (high-priced choice) or in reality placing your satin pillowcase over your normal one at night time time time, then doing away with it all through the day so the mattress suits.

Bonus: It lets in reduce frizzy hair, and will boom shine!

Bonus query from my editor: "I examine that the satin/silk is likewise less absorbent so it permits keep your product on your face, in preference to in the pillowcase. Is this proper or greater internet legend?"

My answer: that is genuine!

What is purging?

Remember the layer of the pores and pores and skin? When a few element is taking walks its way from the basal layer to the stratum corneum (the lowest to the pinnacle) as it's operating its manner up, this is purging.

Sometimes purging happens faster after a expert pores and pores and pores and skin remedy, and that is good enough; it is regular. However, I moreover recognise it can be annoying too, so draw close in there, and recognize that it is healthy on your pores and pores and skin to try this.

What is ice (or bloodless) rolling? Should I be doing that?

Ice rolling is a slight shape of cryotherapy for the pores and pores and skin. It allows carry blood go with the flow to the area, pass lymph fluid, and decrease puffiness,

Some human beings love the sensation of bloodless on their pores and pores and skin (sign me up!) and others do now not. With that in mind, in case you expect you may find it irresistible, pass for it. If you do not, you don't need to each! If you purchase a chilly roller and decide it is not for you, then you could constantly use it on sore muscle organizations so it isn't always a total loss.

What the heck is slugging? It sounds terrible.

I don't disagree with you – I need to truly skip for a contemporary nickname for this.

Slugging is the use of a layer of petroleum jelly or each different ointment-kind product over your one of a kind merchandise at night time time. This offers an occlusive layer that seals the whole thing in. To be a hundred% clear, it does not upload moisture; it lets in other materials to be sealed in or presents a defensive layer.

So with that during mind, the take a look at-up query is, is it ok to do to my pores and pores and pores and skin?

I in reality do no longer sincerely disagree with slugging as an entire, but I do not endorse it massive-strokes style both.

My favored use for this "slugging" (despite the fact that seriously, I want to offer you a modern day name due to the fact this one grosses me out) is for at the same time as a) any character's pores and skin could be very dry or sensitive and we can not get a grip on their moisture barrier, or b) while a person is planning to be outdoor in a dry weather weather (like if they are going snowboarding or some factor like that).

My advice, but, isn't always to use this with a few element that is exfoliating your pores and pores and skin. You do now not need to seal in an enzyme or an acid that could probably over-prompt if stuck in an environment with out somewhere to evaporate off to. If further research suggests otherwise, I'll be happy to eat crow, however as of the time of writing this e-book, I expect it is high-quality to stay with hydrating merchandise handiest under the slugging.

Do I need to put on SPF as quickly as I'm interior? I take a seat down down at a table all day.

Yes, one hundred% certain. If you're going outdoor the least bit, going to be close to a window in any respect, to your automobile or strolling to the mailbox, taking walks your dog, or performing some thing that includes being capable of see mild from out of doors, you want to be carrying sunscreen.

The reason for that is that a few UVA and UVB rays are blocked through the use of a window, however no longer they all. When we're searching on the shape of rays that age the pores and skin - the UVA rays - those ones penetrate the window greater than the UVB rays. So you honestly need to be sporting sunscreen to save you symptoms and symptoms of growing older.

Whether it's miles iciness, fall, spring, summer time or whether or no longer you are indoors or out of doors, you want that protection each day to save you getting old, save you pores and skin cancer, and keep your skin inside the exceptional situation viable for the longest time body.

My makeup has sunscreen in it, so I don't want to apply sunscreen apart from that, right?

No. Wrong. You do need to place on sunscreen beneath that makeup. The possibility of you making use of sufficient makeup to offer right insurance on your pores and pores and skin is slim to none. Put at the sunscreen, then your make-up. Your destiny self thank you you.

How can I maintain products which can be in a jar sanitary?

You can hold your product in jars as sanitary as possible with the resource of washing your palms earlier than you dip your finger in, or possibly better, the usage of a piece scoop or device that may be washed after each use. This will prevent the switch of bacteria to and fro among your fingers or face and the tub.

What even is a facial?

A conventional facial is usually:

• A deep cleanse

• A pores and pores and skin analysis

• Some form of exfoliation - whether or not it's far chemical or manual

• A facial rub down

• Sometimes scalp and/or hand rubdown

• A remedy mask relying on your pores and skin type

• Followed via your finishing products like moisturizer and serum, SPF, that form of element

However, depending in your esthetician, the pattern can also want to trade, the topics executed may want to exchange, and masses of others. If you're looking into going for walks with an esthetician, I endorse that you each look on their internet internet site online to peer in the event that they have an define or call the salon and ask to analyze more approximately the offerings you're interested by.

How regularly want to I get a facial?

I propose a facial at the least one time consistent with month. This ensures that we keep to assemble consequences on your pores and pores and skin and offers you the delivered gain of getting a expert see your pores and pores and skin to help regulate your habitual as wanted. In Europe, it's commonplace for humans to get a facial each unmarried month. Skincare offerings are regarded as form of lengthy-time period care and upkeep, as opposed to in the U.S. Wherein we usually wait until our skin is "appearing up" in advance than working with an esthetician. A lot of troubles can be

47

avoided, or fast resolved with the aid of approach of having normal facials

Can I simply use a mask in location of coming to appearance you every month?

Sure. You can. But sheet mask and domestic treatment mask are truely made to be greater of a protection step amongst facials than a alternative for professional exfoliation, extraction, and treatment.

Think of it like going to the gymnasium. You bypass see a instructor as soon as consistent with week, however you still have to exercising a few instances among seeing them to virtually get consequences, right? So you skip see your esthetician "instructor" as soon as a month and do the upkeep "exercises" with at-home mask and your each day domestic care habitual in among schooling.

Who are chemical peels right for?

Everyone can benefit from a sequence of chemical peels. It's surely approximately making sure which you're getting the right remedy for you. Start slow and coffee and work as a amazing deal as a few issue stronger and your pores and pores and skin might be better prepared to deal with a deeper peel with little to no downtime or real infection.

Why does my esthetician most effective propose the products of their spa?

I'm SO happy you asked! Think of it this manner, we're professionals in the products that we supply and, in preferred, we are able to pleasant advise matters that we understand the most approximately if we want to have integrity. I realize about and clearly believe in, the products that I deliver; consequently, I can with a piece of good fortune suggest those products to my clients, period.

Why doesn't my esthetician extract every breakout spot on my face?

Oh, I love this question; that is this form of correct one. The purpose your esthi won't extract the whole thing is that in the occasion that they extract a few problem that isn't always geared up to pop out, they may motive more damage via bursting the follicle wall and spreading the micro organism round or motive eternal pigmentation marks or scarring. So, they will pick not to extract some thing as it's now not quite geared up to come out.

What are the specific strategies of extraction and that is nice for my pores and skin?

First, let's undergo the brilliant methods extractions are finished:

• Some estheticians do them with gloved arms.

• Some human beings use Q-pointers.

• Some human beings use an extractor device.

• Some human beings use an ultrasonic spatula.

There are many exceptional strategies to do extractions, and it's not constantly that one is better than another for anyone especially. It's more of some thing your esthetician is expert in and what your skin responds nicely to, AKA whether or not or not or not it is releasing the blackheads and blemishes without trouble.

Some states may not allow the use of steel system, so within the ones states, esthi's might not be the usage of an extractor. Some states allow one-of-a-kind tiers of estheticians to apply lancets to extract and unique ranges cannot. Some states do now not allow the usage of lancets the least bit.

So there can be loads of factors that pass into this. The splendid problem is virtually to recognise that you most effective want to have extractions carried out on topics which may be organized to be extracted via a professional esthetician who is privy to how a ways to transport and on the equal time as to prevent.

Can I extract acne at home?

No. And positive. (I realize you like it as quickly as I say that, right?!)

The fantastic acne which I provide my seal of reputation of my clients extract on their non-public are the ones that have a white head in the middle. So believe the pimple that has a crimson ring, and a white raised middle.

Here are the stairs to well extracting at domestic:

• Wash your palms very well.

• Using a lancet, gently poke one hole in the middle of the white spot of the pimple. This could be very vital because it offers the pus, sebum, and micro organism somewhere to go out.

• Using two cotton swabs, lightly push across the purple ring, utilising moderate stress downward and up from beneath. You will see the white pus, in all likelihood some green, or yellow, or even a tiny bit of blood come out of the spot you poked a hollow in.

• If topics do now not come out...DO NOT FORCE IT. Wait an afternoon or and strive yet again, but don't forget, be mild; you do no longer want to stress some factor.

• You also can have a take a look at a few slight stress or an ice dice to carry down swelling and prevent any bleeding, but for the love of God, do not select.

Does hair on my face growth decrease lower back thicker if I wax?

No, the hair for your face does no longer expand lower back thicker or darker if you shave or wax it. Vellus hairs, the little blonde "peach fuzz" that is on many human beings's faces, isn't hormone-related hair so it will extend over again the identical. Sometimes at the same time as the hair grows decrease lower back in, it feels blunter, and with that, it is able to sense like it's thicker however it is truely now not. If you're getting a dermablade remedy or shaving your face, it simply is while you'll be maximum probably to enjoy the blunt-feeling hairs. If you're waxing, the hair is pulled out from the root, so it's far more likely to revel in softer because it grows again in. If you do enjoy darker, coarser hairs growing in, the ones are from a hormone exchange. Unfortunately, pulling them out does not make them expand again more finely.

Chapter 6: What ought to I avoid before waxing?

Three to seven days earlier than waxing, you are going to need to keep away from retinol or exfoliating products so that you can sensitize or thin your pores and skin.

A phrase to take very considerably: in case you are on Accutane, you have to no longer wax in any respect for the time you are on it. You'll want to be tweezed or threaded for facial hair removal, and shave for any preferred body hair elimination.

Why does a few pores and skin care ruin my towels?

It might be due to one in every of things: both you used a staining object and the towel wasn't washed or dealt with nicely (dark-coloured skin care mask for instance) in any other case you used a product with benzoyl peroxide in it, a superb manner to bleach your towels.

I advocate having a hard and fast of seven face towels which you use first-class for your face and best one an afternoon each. Get ones which you do now not thoughts bleaching or staining.

My skin is breaking out….Help!!!

There are such loads of factors that would cause this, however we're capable of start with some easy questions on way of life:

• When you shower, do you wash your hair or your face first? Always wash your face closing so you can do away with any buildup from conditioner at the pores and skin. Better but, wash outdoor of the shower; the bathe temp is simply too warm in your face.

• Do you parent out often? If so, are you washing your face after?

• Do you play sports sports in which helmets are required? Are you disinfecting it in advance than placing your face interior?

• Are you changing your pillowcase as a minimum as soon as every week? Are you converting your face towel every day?

• Are you disinfecting your cell smartphone regularly? If you are at the cellphone at artwork, is that one getting wiped easy?

• What is your eating regimen like?

• Have you been getting sufficient water?

• What's your strain diploma like?

• Have you lately changed or gotten off begin manipulate?

• Are you close to your period?

I should float on and on, the ones are sincerely a number of the elements that could cause breakouts, and we want to appearance decrease returned about 60-ninety days to appearance in which a number of the ones elements might in all likelihood come into play. So, for the sake of time, I can't answer your particular pores and pores and skin needs, however I can will will let you know how I might also need to deal with my pores and pores and pores and skin while it breaks out:

I begin via manner of going decrease again to fundamentals thru making sure I'm cleaning well, now not getting lazy with wiping down my cellular smartphone, converting face towels and sheets, and getting enough water.

Next, I think through my each day ordinary. Is there someplace that some factor is touching my face in any respect? Is that problem cleaned often?

What is my stress diploma like? Can I begin to consciousness on reducing pressure if it is excessive? What does that seem like?

Is my weight loss plan healthful? Or have I been pressure ingesting? (Yes, I try this. I'm human y'all.)

Next, I deal with my product picks. If I even have not changed something in recent times, I can rule that out.

Then I make certain to cope with the regions wished with glycolic and salicylic acid, benzoyl peroxide on the equal time as wished, and breakout patches. (Also, remember at the same time as the usage of benzoyl peroxide, use best white towels and sheets and stuff you do now not thoughts bleaching out.)

Why is my pores and pores and pores and skin dry and breaking out?

Our pores and skin is constantly looking for an equilibrium of water and oil. In this case, your pores and pores and skin is likely overproducing oil to seize up on dehydration. P. Acnes micro organism feed on the sebum (oily count number) on our pores and pores and pores and skin, so whilst we are overproducing oil to catch up on the dryness, the P. Acnes get a snack, which then reasons more breakouts.

In this case, I usually suggest up your consumption of water, prevent result, and greens, and to feature a hyaluronic acid serum to your habitual to feature hydration into the pores and pores and skin and help it regain a better balance.

How can I lessen decrease back my pores?

You're not going to like me for this, but you purchased this ebook to get the no-nonsense no-bullsh*t solutions on your questions. So right here it's far. Unfortunately, there is no real manner to decrease your pores due to the fact they're now not muscular tissues.

The proper information is, the cleaner you're pores are, the smaller they will appearance. Using a cleaning tool with an ultrasonic cleaning opportunity will assist to make certain that your pores stay as smooth as feasible.

Why don't you advise the use of coconut oil on the face?

I used to notably propose coconut oil as a pre-cleanse step. However, as I discovered out greater about pores and skin, I observed out that some human beings can use coconut oil on their pores and pores and skin and different humans cannot. The motive for this is, coconut oil may be comedogenic for a few human beings. On the comedogenic scale (which measures how possibly a few component is to clog your pores) coconut oil falls quite excessive because of this that it is much more likely to clog pores, specifically in humans who have acne. Some humans will don't have any trouble with it in any respect! But because of the reality that extra people than no longer may want to have problems, I don't generally suggest it to be used to your face anymore.

So wherein can you operate coconut oil? It is a exceptional body moisturizer, in case you aren't at risk of body zits. It's moreover notable as a hair remedy, so long as you wash it out previous to washing your face.

What should I endorse if you preferred to feature an oil into your regular that could be a top notch deal much much less comedogenic? Jojoba oil, pink raspberry leaf oil, sea buckthorn oil, and hemp seed oil. All of those are tremendous at the pores and pores and pores and skin. Seek out right remarkable cold-pressed oils and upload a drop for your moisturizer or study over your moisturizer at night time for tremendous effects. You can also use the oils as a pre-cleanse to interrupt down make-up and debris on the pores and pores and pores and skin earlier than using your cleanser to easy it all away.

How do I use retinol?

If you are a novice to retinol use, you can have heard it could be sincerely disturbing or drying. This is sincerely authentic for some people! To keep away from as an lousy lot inflammation as feasible, I usually recommend you begin with retinol one time each week for a month.

If your pores and pores and pores and skin has adjusted nicely, you can skip up to 2 times each week for the subsequent month.

If your pores and pores and skin has once more adjusted well, you may bypass up to a few times regular with week for the following month. (And so on, operating as an awful lot as every night time time time if desired, and if your pores and pores and skin can tolerate it.)

Some people will prevent at one to two instances every week, and this is ideal enough! Other people will cross on and be able to use it each unmarried night time time time; it truely is based upon on how touchy and reactive your skin is and what percentage of various sorts of exfoliants you're the use of.

What is walnut scrub properly for?

What is it notable for? Honestly, it is definitely correct as a foot and leg scrub. The pores and pores and skin on our feet is the thickest on our frame, so it's far sincerely right for that. However, I could not use it - or advocate it - to be used anywhere else. The floor-up walnut shells and walnut portions are too tough and jagged to use in your face, in which the pores and pores and skin is the thinnest on our our our our bodies. It can cause micro-tears within the surface of the pores and pores and pores and skin, that have the potential to spread bacteria or cause brilliant infection to touchy pores and skin or maybe motive sensitivity in formerly non-indignant pores and skin.

Stick to using walnuts leg or foot scrubbing and you'll be right to move.

Are alcohols in skin care horrific?

Some are, and some aren't. There is a form of alcohol called a fatty alcohol which includes such things as acetyl, cetyl, isostearyl or cetearyl alcohol which may be perfectly pleasant for the pores and pores and pores and skin. They're honestly appropriate for dry pores and skin. However, in case you ever see a product categorised with SD or isopropyl alcohol, those materials are not desirable in your pores and skin, they may be too drying to use frequently, and will reason damage in your pores and pores and skin's barrier function.

Should I put on a mineral or chemical sunscreen? Does it depend?

Honestly, wearing sunscreen at all is in truth the maximum vital element if we are without a doubt talking sunscreen as an entire. If, however, you are involved about any of it stepping into your bloodstream for any motive, I ought to advise a mineral sunscreen. Mineral sunscreens are ones with zinc oxide or titanium oxide as their active substances. Chemical sunscreens have oxybenzone, avobenzone, octisalate, and lots of others as their energetic elements.

As of the time of scripting this e-book (past due 2020), sunscreens are within the way of assessment thru the FDA. Studies have placed that a number of the materials can get into the bloodstream; however, they have got not determined if those components are dangerous inside the bloodstream or in truth are present there.

With that being said, in case you are concerned approximately that, I may want to hold on with mineral sunscreens inside the meantime. Mineral sunscreens became as quickly as exceptional thick, opaque method that felt sticky at the pores and pores and skin. Over the years, the beauty beauty (AKA the feel, texture) of those products has become very state-of-the-art.

What are peptides?

Peptides are small chains of amino acids that paintings collectively to assemble topics or sign subjects to appear in the pores and pores and skin. When or extra peptides are mixed, they devise proteins, that are the building blocks of the whole lot in our pores and pores and pores and skin. They are essentially the vendors to create notable exchange within the pores and pores and pores and skin.

CHAPTER 7: Understanding Your Skin Type

In order to have healthful, glowing pores and skin, you want to recognize your pores and pores and skin type. Your skin type will determine the varieties of products and wearing activities a superb way to work super for you. This bankruptcy will talk the particular types of pores and pores and skin, which consist of regular, oily, dry, combination, and touchy. You will discover ways to pick out out your pores and skin kind and what products and workouts are outstanding ideal for each type.

Understanding your pores and skin type is an important step to carrying out wholesome, sparkling pores and pores and skin. It can be difficult to choose out your pores and pores and skin type, however it's miles essential to acquire this so that it will make certain you're the usage of the proper merchandise and taking the right steps to care for your pores and pores and skin.

Skin sorts are typically damaged down into 4 training: oily, dry, aggregate, and touchy. Oily pores and skin is vulnerable to shine, enlarged pores, and breakouts. Dry pores and pores and pores and skin is frequently characterized thru flaking, itching, and tightness. Combination pores and skin is a mixture of each oily and dry pores and pores and skin, with an oily T-quarter (forehead, nose, and chin) and dry patches somewhere else. Sensitive pores and pores and skin is at risk of redness and infection, and is with out problem angry by using products with fragrances or harsh additives.

The nice manner to pick out out out your pores and pores and skin type is to assess it over numerous days or perhaps weeks. Pay interest to the manner your pores and pores and pores and skin appears and feels while you awaken in the morning, when you cleanse your face, and throughout the day. Notice any areas that will be inclined to be oilier or drier than others, and the way your pores and skin responds to exceptional products.

It's additionally critical to look at that pores and pores and skin kind can change over the years. As we age, our pores and pores and skin tends to become drier, so it's crucial to re-observe your pores and pores and skin kind on a everyday basis. Factors together with way of life, healthy dietweight-reduction plan, and the surroundings can also have an impact for your pores and pores and skin type.

Once you've diagnosed your skin kind, you can take steps to ensure you're giving your pores and pores and skin the care it wishes. Oily skin will gain from merchandise that absorb oil and unclog pores, at the same time as dry skin wishes moisturizers and gentle cleansers. Combination pores and pores and skin want to use merchandise that target every oily and dry areas, which includes oil-loose moisturizers. Sensitive pores and pores and skin should use products which might be free of fragrances and vicious materials.

Understanding your pores and pores and skin kind is step one to carrying out healthful, glowing pores and pores and pores and skin. Identifying your pores and pores and skin kind will assist you choose the proper merchandise and growth the outstanding pores and skin care routine in your particular wishes.

CHAPTER 8: The Benefits of a Good Skin Care Routine

Having an amazing pores and skin care everyday is critical for retaining wholesome and younger looking pores and skin. Skin care isn't pretty much using merchandise, it's miles approximately know-how your pores and skin kind and desires and following a ordinary habitual to preserve your pores and pores and skin within the pleasant scenario possible. There are many unique components to a brilliant pores and skin care routine, and each one is critical to your substantial pores and pores and skin health.

Cleansing

Cleansing is an vital part of pores and pores and skin care and should be achieved at the least as quick as a day, preferably two times. Cleansing permits to remove dust, oil, and other impurities from the pores and pores and skin, leaving it feeling clean and refreshed. It is crucial to pick a cleaner this is appropriate for your pores and skin kind and to use it lightly, as harsh scrubbing can harm the pores and pores and skin.

Cleansers

The form of cleanser you use is critical in your skin care ordinary. There are many specific kinds of cleansers available, beginning from foaming cleansers to oils and balms. It is vital to choose out a cleanser that is suitable for your pores and skin type and to apply it gently.

Exfoliation

Exfoliation is an essential part of a first rate skin care normal and have to be done instances in line with week. Exfoliation permits to cast off vain pores and pores and skin cells, unclog pores, and display the sparkling, healthful pores and pores and skin below. There are many awesome forms of exfoliants available, starting from bodily scrubs to chemical exfoliants. It is vital to choose an exfoliant this is suitable to your pores and skin type.

Moisturizing

Moisturizing is an vital a part of pores and pores and skin care, because it allows to preserve the skin hydrated and looking healthful. It is crucial to pick out out a moisturizer that is appropriate to your pores and skin type and to use it after cleansing and exfoliating. It is also crucial to use moisturizer at a few diploma in the day, mainly after showering or swimming.

Moisturizers

Just like cleansers, there are many one in every of a type sorts of moisturizers to be had, beginning from slight creams to heavy creams. It is crucial to choose a moisturizer this is suitable in your pores and pores and pores and skin type and to apply it after cleaning and exfoliating.

Sun Protection

Sun safety is important for wholesome pores and pores and skin, due to the fact the sun's UV rays can cause harm to the pores and skin, main to premature developing older, sunburn, and even pores and pores and skin maximum cancers. It is vital to wear a full-size-spectrum sunscreen each day, even on cloudy days, as the solar's rays can despite the fact that penetrate the clouds. Sunscreen need to be reapplied every hours and after swimming or sweating.

By following an top notch pores and pores and skin care normal, you could keep your pores and pores and pores and skin searching wholesome and extra youthful. It is critical to understand your pores and pores and pores and skin kind and desires and to select merchandise which may be appropriate on your pores and pores and skin. Additionally, it's far vital to put on sunscreen each day and to reapply it regularly. Following the ones steps can help to keep your pores and pores and skin wholesome and searching its first-rate.

CHAPTER 9: Self-Care

Self-care is the exercise of taking an energetic feature in shielding one's very very own well-being and happiness, specifically at some stage in times of strain. It can contain sports activities inclusive of eating wholesome, getting enough sleep, exercising, taking time for yourself, and engaging in sports that bring joy and relaxation. Self-care is an critical part of common intellectual fitness, and may help to prevent burnout and depression.

When it includes growing a self-care recurring, it's essential to first understand what your desires are. Everyone has splendid dreams close to looking after themselves, so it's important to make an effort to choose out out what's most crucial to you. Once you have were given recognized your desires, it's vital to make a plan to fulfill them. This need to contain putting aside time every day to interact in sports activities that make you sense correct, which include taking a walk, reading a e-book, or task a hobby.

It's additionally crucial to take note of your bodily health. Eating a balanced healthy dietweight-reduction plan, getting enough sleep, and appealing in regular exercise can assist to preserve your body healthy and your thoughts clean. If you are suffering to make healthful choices, it is able to be useful to enlist the help of a nutritionist or private teacher.

It's additionally important to take time for yourself. This want to contain taking time to lighten up, meditate, or have interaction in sports which you enjoy. Taking time for your self can help to lessen stress and save you burnout.

Finally, it's critical to workout self-compassion. This consists of being kind and records to yourself, even whilst you make errors or face hard situations. Practicing self-compassion can help to enhance your highbrow health and growth your commonplace sense of properly being.

Self-care is an crucial a part of typical highbrow fitness. Taking the time to discover your needs and increase a plan to meet them can assist to save you burnout and despair, and may assist to increase it slow-honored feel of nicely-being.

Stress Management

Stress can also want to have a big impact on our bodily and intellectual fitness, and dealing with it's far vital for regular wellness. Skin care can be a superb manner to lessen pressure and beautify your temper, it is why it's so essential to make the effort to take care of your skin.

When it involves stress manipulate, one of the first steps is to apprehend and extensively recognized the property of your strain. This can include work, circle of relatives, relationships, fee variety, and extremely good duties. Once you've diagnosed the resources of your pressure, you may start to develop techniques to higher deal with them.

One of the satisfactory methods to manipulate stress is thru rest and self-care. Take time to do sports activities that make you sense snug, which encompass yoga, meditation, and deep respiration physical sports. Spend time exterior and playing nature. Connect with friends and circle of relatives and make sure to take breaks in some unspecified time in the future of the day.

When it involves pores and pores and pores and skin care, the most important detail is to guard your pores and pores and skin from the solar. Wear sunscreen and hats even as outside, and use a moisturizer that is proper to your pores and skin kind. Make sure to smooth your face twice a day, and use a slight cleaner that acquired't strip away natural oils. Exfoliate as soon as in line with week to get rid of lifeless pores and pores and skin cells and keep your pores and skin looking smooth.

Finally, don't forget about to drink plenty of water. Water permits to flush out pollution and keep your pores and pores and skin hydrated. Eating a balanced eating regimen with plenty of give up result and greens is likewise important for skin fitness.

Stress manage and skin care move hand-in-hand. When you contend with yourself, you're looking after your pores and pores and skin. Taking the time to prioritize your health, each physical and intellectual, is essential for everyday well being.

Diet and Nutrition

Diet and vitamins performs a important position in pores and pores and skin care. Eating a wholesome, balanced food regimen that is high in vitamins, minerals, antioxidants, and other important nutrients is the vital factor to maintaining wholesome, younger pores and pores and skin. Eating a whole lot of surrender result and vegetables, lean proteins, and healthful fat is essential for pores and pores and skin health.

Fruits and veggies provide the body with important nutrients, minerals, and antioxidants. These nutrients help to resource healthy mobile growth and regeneration, it's critical for healthful, glowing pores and skin. Fruits and greens also are immoderate in fiber, which permits to keep the digestive tool strolling effortlessly and might assist reduce contamination. Eating numerous coloured end result and greens inclusive of oranges, berries, spinach, and broccoli can assist make sure you are getting a variety of nutrients and minerals to assist pores and pores and pores and skin health.

Protein is an crucial macronutrient for pores and pores and skin fitness. Protein allows to sell collagen manufacturing and may help reduce wrinkles. It moreover enables to maintain strong and healthful hair and nails. Lean proteins which includes chicken, fish, eggs, and beans are exceptional assets of protein.

Healthy fat are important for skin health as they help to maintain the pores and pores and skin hydrated and plump. Healthy assets of fat include nuts, avocados, olive oil, and salmon.

In addition to healthy ingesting, eating loads of water is essential for wholesome pores and pores and skin. Water enables to hold the pores and pores and skin hydrated and may assist flush out pollutants. It is critical to drink at least 8 glasses of water steady with day to make certain your pores and pores and skin is getting the hydration it desires.

Overall, food plan and nutrients plays an critical position in pores and pores and skin care. Eating a balanced weight loss plan this is excessive in vitamins, minerals, antioxidants, and different important vitamins is vital for wholesome, more younger pores and pores and pores and skin. Eating some of surrender result and veggies, lean proteins, and healthful fats, and consuming lots of water can assist hold your pores and pores and skin searching and feeling its exquisite.

In addition to ingesting a healthy, balanced healthy dietweight-reduction plan, it's also vital to apply great pores and skin care merchandise. Using products with natural components can assist to guard and nourish the pores and skin. Applying sunscreen is also crucial for preventing solar harm and pores and pores and skin most cancers. Finally, getting everyday exercising, avoiding smoking, and handling pressure can all help to promote healthy, glowing pores and skin.

CHAPTER 10: Professional Skin Care

Skin care is an important a part of fashionable health and well being, and expert skin care is a critical step in attaining healthy and fantastic pores and skin. Professional pores and skin care is the exercise of being involved for the skin with professional techniques and merchandise to keep and improve its look. Professional pores and skin care remedies and products can assist to reduce the signs and symptoms of having antique, improve the arrival of pores and skin, and prevent and deal with high-quality pores and skin situations.

At the coronary coronary coronary heart of professional pores and skin care is right skin care strategies and products. The use of the proper pores and pores and skin care products and techniques is essential for attaining healthy and wonderful pores and skin. Professional pores and skin care merchandise are mainly formulated to cope with the desires of diverse pores and skin kinds, and they will be frequently an lousy lot extra powerful than over the counter products. Professional pores and pores and skin care treatments also are to be had to enhance the appearance and feel of the pores and pores and skin, and to deal with unique skin situations.

Professional pores and skin care remedies generally incorporate the usage of specialised equipment and products to exfoliate, cleanse, and nourish the pores and skin. Facials, peels, and microdermabrasion are a number of the maximum well-known expert skin care treatments. Facials involve using cleansers, exfoliants, and moisturizers to deeply cleanse and nourish the pores and skin, whilst peels and microdermabrasion are used to exfoliate and do away with the top layer of dull pores and skin cells.

In addition to professional skin care remedies, professional pores and skin care products are also used to address particular skin troubles. Professional pores and skin care products are often more potent than over-the-counter merchandise and can be used to address acne, dark spots, wrinkles, and specific pores and pores and skin troubles. Professional pores and pores and pores and skin care products furthermore generally comprise higher concentrations of lively factors, that might assist to decorate the appearance and feel of the pores and skin.

Professional skin care is an crucial a part of widespread health and fitness, and it is able to assist to beautify the advent and revel in of the skin. By using the proper skin care products and remedies, you can acquire wholesome and brilliant pores and skin.

Facials

A facial is a beauty treatment this is designed to easy and revitalize the pores and pores and pores and skin in your face. It normally consists of cleaning, exfoliating, and moisturizing, as well as lots of precise treatments relying on the kind of facial you pick out and the state of affairs of your pores and skin. Facials are a outstanding way to loosen up and enhance your pores and pores and skin's look and fitness.

Benefits of Facials

Facials provide a number of advantages, from enhancing the general look of your pores and skin to offering deep-cleaning and exfoliation, which can help to limit the results of having vintage. Facials can also help to reduce pimples, treatment blemishes, and even out skin tone. Additionally, facials can help to reduce the advent of wrinkles and notable strains, further to offering hydration and nourishment to the pores and pores and skin.

Types of Facials

There are a number of considered one of a kind varieties of facials available, each of which is designed to goal a specific pores and pores and skin scenario. Some of the most well-known sorts of facials encompass:

• Rejuvenating Facial: A rejuvenating facial is designed to decorate the overall appearance and experience of your pores and pores and skin. This form of facial usually consists of cleansing, exfoliation, a mask, and a moisturizer.

• Acne Facial: An zits facial is designed to cope with and save you breakouts at the same time as moreover supporting to clear clogged pores. This form of facial usually includes cleansing, exfoliation, a mask, and a moisturizer.

• Sensitive Skin Facial: A touchy pores and pores and skin facial is designed to assuage and nourish touchy pores and skin. This shape of facial generally consists of cleaning, exfoliation, a masks, and a moisturizer.

• Anti-Aging Facial: An anti-developing antique facial is designed to reduce the visible symptoms and signs and signs and symptoms of developing antique. This form of facial commonly consists of cleaning, exfoliation, a mask, and a moisturizer.

• Detoxifying Facial: A detoxifying facial is designed to rid your pores and pores and skin of impurities and pollution. This form of facial normally consists of cleansing, exfoliation, a masks, and a moisturizer.

How to Prepare for a Facial

Before getting a facial, it's miles vital to make certain that your pores and skin is well prepared. First, you have to make certain to cleanse your pores and pores and skin very well and put off any make-up. It is likewise critical to avoid the use of harsh exfoliants or some extraordinary merchandise that can worsen your pores and pores and skin in advance than your facial. Additionally, it's far crucial to drink hundreds of water and avoid any strenuous interest in advance than your facial, as this will reason your pores and pores and skin to become dehydrated.

Facials are a tremendous manner to relax and decorate the advent and fitness of your pores and pores and skin. There are severa one-of-a-type kinds of facials available, every of that's designed to intention a specific pores and pores and skin assignment. Before getting a facial, it's miles critical to make sure that your pores and pores and skin is properly organized through way of cleansing and heading off any merchandise that could get worse your skin. With the proper education and care, facials can assist to enhance the look and enjoy of your pores and skin.

Chapter 11: Understanding your pores and skin

So masses of us are going out and looking for splendor care products or using make-up with out understanding our pores and pores and skin type. As a result we waste cash on products that do not in form our pores and skin, or worse nonetheless might also furthermore have an negative response to the product resulting in trouble skin.

Your pores and skin kind isn't always going to trade while your pores and pores and skin scenario can change due to the fact it's miles based upon on different factors which incorporates healthy eating plan.

The pores and pores and skin makes up about five% of someone's body weight, it's miles the most important unmarried organ of the human frame. It lets in to guard us in opposition to UV radiation, micro organism and threatening chemical substances. The state of affairs of the pores and skin may be a excellent indication of the manner healthful

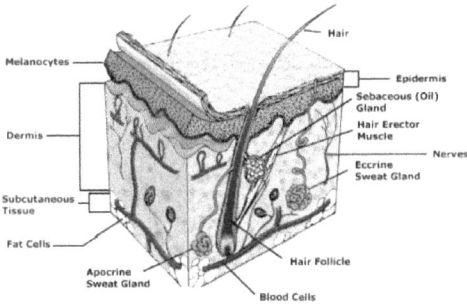

the frame is.

As you can see from the diagram above the pores and pores and skin is usually made from the epidermis, epidermis and subcutaneous.

Skin kinds can be classed into the subsequent 5 classes:

1: Normal Skin

Congratulations in case you are one of the fortunate few who have normal pores and pores and skin. Basically due to this the sebaceous gland (produces oil) produces a substance referred to as sebum at a practical price.

This allows for the pores and pores and skin to appear not oily or dry, looking wet and active. Please word that this pores and skin kind nonetheless advantages from constant

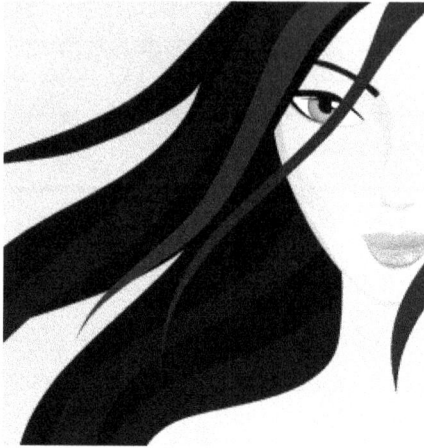

care.

2: Dry Skin

This skin type is due to underperforming oil glands that do not appear to be producing as masses oil due to the fact the pores and skin desires. As a quit end result of this pores and pores and pores and skin specialists take shipping of as true with that this pores and pores and pores and skin kind is most at risk of untimely ageing and as such wishes committed care and hobby to lessen the results.

Dry pores and pores and pores and skin normally seems duller, itchy, patchy, flared up and probably flaky. As the pores and pores and skin lacks moisture from the glands, it desires to be crowned up via everyday eating of water and the good enough pores and skin care merchandise that target tackling dry pores and skin.

Do

- Use cream / paste based make-up

- Drink 1-2 litres of water every day

- Cleanse face with products created for dry pores and pores and pores and skin

- Moisturise with products created for dry pores and pores and skin

Don't

- Use powder / dry make-up

- Stay in the solar too lengthy

- Stay in air conditioned environments too lengthy

3: Oily Skin

Complete contrary of dry pores and skin. The glands produce too much oil, which finally ends up in the pores and pores and pores and skin having more oil than it wishes consequently bringing the oil to the skin's ground making it visible.

The most important advantage of getting oily pores and pores and skin is that people who have it will be predisposed to age higher as wrinkles are delayed or reduced. The disadvantage is that your pores and pores and skin can be vulnerable to blackheads and zits.

Do

- Choose a moisturiser that is created especially for oily pores and pores and skin – sorts

- Use oil unfastened products

- Use powder based definitely make-up

Don't

- Use any glossy merchandise as your skin will sincerely produce that impact

- Over cleanse

4: Sensitive Skin:

This pores and skin type may be either of dry, normal or oily. Sensitive pores and pores and skin is maximum probably to be liable to an allergy to beauty care / make-up merchandise. It can flare up and become itchy reacting to environmental conditions.

Do

- Test makeup or beauty products on a pattern of your skin for a time body in advance than the usage of it extensively

- Use products which have been hypersensitivity tested or u . S . A . 'hypoallergenic'

- Benefits maximum from mild and natural skin care

Don't

- Use products that comprise alcohol & fragrance oils

5: Combination Skin:

This is a mixture of oily and dry pores and pores and skin. The tremendous recommendation can be to trial and errors products that wholesome your pores and pores and pores and skin and look at the recommendation under the headings above that be sincerely proper for you.

Cleanse, Tone & Moisturise

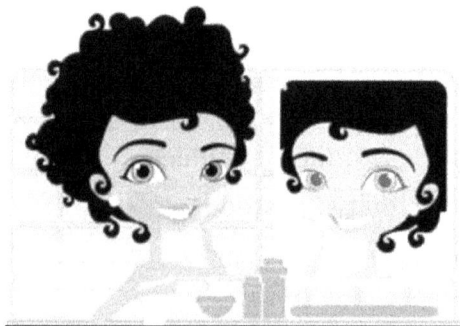

Naturally being worried to your skin is properly up there as one of the most essential matters that you could ever do to save you growing older and searching healthy. Normally, ladies try to cowl up horrible skin care with makeup and surgical treatment. Stress and weather can also have an impact on the situation of the pores and pores and pores and skin.

As a fundamental if you do the following you will be on the street to having appealing and healthy pores and skin.

1: Cleansing

Cleansing skin is a demand for truly all people regardless of whether or not or now not they use make up, specifically because of the truth skin draws loads of dirt at some point of the day and this could live at the pores and skin besides dealt with with a cleanser.

By cleansing your pores and pores and pores and skin earlier than you exercising makeup it's going to come up with a clean face to artwork and a clean face earlier than you nod off.

The trick with cleansers is to recognize your pores and pores and skin kind earlier than you purchase one, if you have touchy pores and skin make truly positive you buy a milder cleanser than the norm.

Steps

1: Wash arms; get rid of mascara and eye shadow with eye make-up remover

2: Pour some cleanser into the palm of your hand and dab it over the face (cheeks, nose, forehead and chin) with wonderful hand.

3: Spread cleaner via massaging into the pores and pores and skin in an upward and outward motion (don't stretch pores and skin)

four: Remove the purifier with tissue pads / cotton pads or water lightly the usage of upward and outward motion

2: Toning

Toning lets in do away with extra oil from your pores and pores and skin, it can moreover assist refresh skin and upload glow for your face.

It continues to be debated inside the pores and skin care enterprise company on whether firming is to be accomplished each day, I assume the answer is everybody is wonderful and if it fits then you definately use it regular if no longer transfer to every distinct day.

Note: The more chemical loose your toner is, the extra herbal and higher to your pores and skin.

Depending on the shape of toner: can also want to every spray on or pat on with cotton / tissue pads

3: Moisturise

Moisturiser is like feeding your thirsty pores and skin. The most vital issue is to recognize the kind of pores and skin you've got earlier than you rush out to buy a present day-day moisturiser.

There are hundreds of moisturisers out in the marketplace in recent times so please do your research in advance than parting with your money, sincerely because of the fact a movie star or model uses a moisturiser doesn't advise it is going to fit your pores and pores and skin too.

If you have oily skin then try no longer to purchase a moisturiser containing too much petroleum jelly / oils as this will make your pores and skin look even more oily.

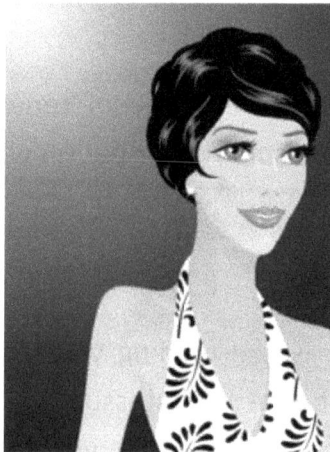

Steps:

1: Apply moderate quantities of moisturiser on your face via first of all dabbing it onto your brow, nostril, cheeks and chin.

2: Work into skin in upward and outward motions till it fades into the pores and pores and skin

3: Reapply to any regions that require it

Chapter 12: Makeup Tools

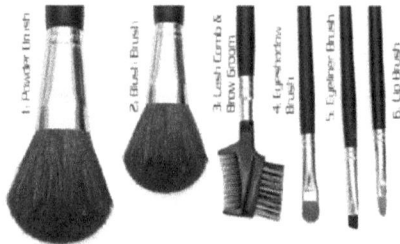

So many brushes! Confused? Well don't be, I actually have tried to offer an reason at the back of the motive of every of the pictured make-up equipment in brief under.

1: Powder Brush

Generally used to dirt powder onto the face usually after foundation to offer a matte give up

Tips

- Only use a top notch great brush because the end may possibly understate all of your guidance make-up software program

- Use a medium sized brush

- Ask a makeup counter if you could use it on your pores and pores and skin in advance than buy

2: Blush Brush

You guessed it, used to use blusher

Tips

- Not too massive and now not too small! But certainly proper. If it's far too large you risk utilising it to a much broader area than intended. Too small and you will be stricken by manner of constructing up of product on your software

- Should be more impregnable than the powder brush. Ask a makeup counter if you can use it on your pores and pores and pores and skin earlier than buy

three: Lash Comb & Brow Groom

Can remedy mascara build up via way of combing through; also can ensure even distribution of mascara. The brush side is used really to neaten up the brow vicinity. You also can get the ones in separate brushes in preference to a combined.

Tips

- Makeup artists will be inclined to apply in a slower movement than once they workout mascara

4: Eyeshadow Brush

Used to apply eyeshadow over the whole eyelid or throughout the rim of the attention location.

Tips

- It is pretty commonplace to have a couple of type of eyeshadow brush as they come in various sizes and interest

- Concentrated: Applied across the rim of the eyes

- Softer: Application over the eyelid

five: Eyeliner Brush

Used to cautiously spread eyeliner, the brush allows for differing styles counting on the pressure achieved to the brush.

Tips

- Thinner Application: Use brush gently (high-quality tipped brush)

- Thicker Application: press a touch more firmly this will spread the bristles and a make a far broader line

- More drastically used with liquid merchandise

6: Lip Brush

Used to in reality add definition to the lips

Tips

- To accentuate the easy lip line you may want a flat brush

- The technique and the thoughts-set you exercise the lipstick may want to have a massive impact on the general effect

Facial Structures

There are many facial systems that a makeup artist desires to recognize, that is simply so the makeup software program can be tailor-made to maximize on the face shape and favored fashion.

Below are the essential difficulty facial systems a makeup artist want to be privy to:

Square Face:

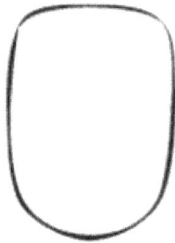

- Similar to spherical face but sharper edges

- Apply darker foundation on each cheeks and forehead

- Use lighter basis at the chin

- Apply blusher to the apples of your cheeks in a rounded sample mixed properly

Long Face:

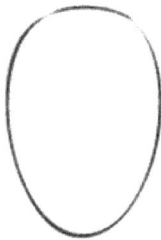

- Raised forehead and distinctive jawline

- Darker foundation on forehead and chin area

- Ensure blusher doesn't benefit the outer corners of the attention or the lower tip of the nostril place

 Round Face:

- Apply darker foundation on every cheeks however place a mild colour on your chin place

- Place blusher on the cheek bones and perspective the coloration up in a instantly line

Oval Face:

- Ideal face form and perfectly symmetrical

- Supports maximum make-up dispositions

- Minimal contouring required

Chapter 13: Highlighting & Shading

You can draw interest to or away from a place with the use of powerful highlighting and shading techniques. A makeup artist can use matte tones to coloration a place or shimmer/matte tones for highlighting. Shading pushes once more a place with highlighting brings it in advance.

Foundation Base Application

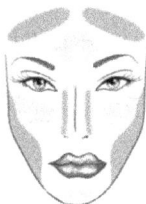

Shading:
> Hairline Area
> Temple area
> Eye Crease
> Hollow cheek areas
> Sides and tip of nose
> Under chin and neck

Highlighting:
> Forehead
> Brow Bone
> Eye lid centre
> Under Eye
> Cheek Bone
> Nose Centre
> Upper Lip
> Chin Centre

There are a few elements that make the difference among an terrific natural searching foundation software and a horrible one. Bad ones have a tendency to be wherein people can manifestly study which you have used foundation, in particular because of incorrect basis shade or lack of mixing into your pores and pores and skin.

Follow those smooth steps and be at the manner to perfecting your basis make up software.

Steps:

1: Moisturise (Important)

2: Dot some basis to your face: brow, chin, cheeks, neck and nose

three: Either the usage of your fingertips or a basis brush BLEND all the foundation into your pores and skin ensuring a terrific spread, till the foundation colour seems like your herbal skin shade

Tips:

- It can help to use fingertips for the inspiration mixing technique

- Some foundations require a mild software of powder to set well, wherein case observe a pleasant first-class translucent powder evenly over the face the use of a powder brush

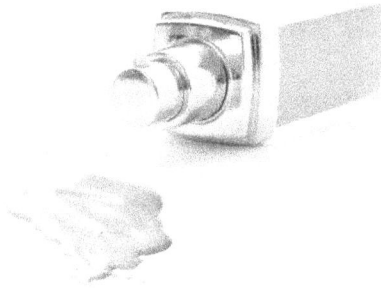

Eye – Shading & Blending

By using eye shadow especially colours and textures you may melt or accentuate your appearance. Create a high quality temper or maybe beautify your eye shape counting on the appearance which you need to reap.

Step 1:

Apply concealer gently over the top eye lid

Step 2:

Apply base paint and set with translucent powder to the pinnacle eye lid

Step three:

Apply a lighter colour of eye shadow to the whole pinnacle eye lid with a flat eye shadow

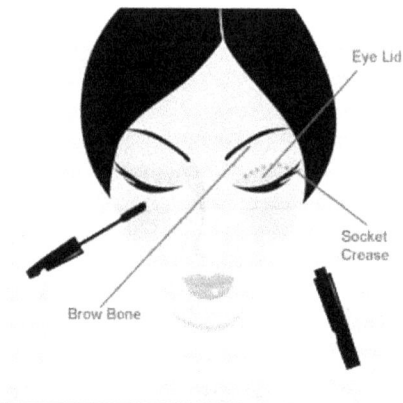

brush

Step four:

With a darker color of eye shadow, examine to the socket crease place with flat brush – make certain which you mixture frivolously with a mixing brush (exercise the darkish shadow at the outer nook of the eye in a horizontal "V" shape).

Step five:

Apply highlighter to the brow bone and the inner nook of the attention using a flat brush.

Eye Liner

Make up artists have a tendency to apply eye liner on customers to feature a glance of class and wow element. It may be hard to get the cling of it for self software program, but as with the whole thing, guidance makes best and the outcomes are remarkable.

1: Wink: During self software program application you'll want to keep one eye open and the possibility one (software program eye) as closed

2: The Line: Eye liner is to be accomplished at the foundation of the top lash as showed, when you have problem drawing a line in a single bypass the draw a dotted line after which be a part of up the dots as verified via the usage of the picture underneath

three: Keep going over this line till it's miles a regular duration and the thickness you need to go for

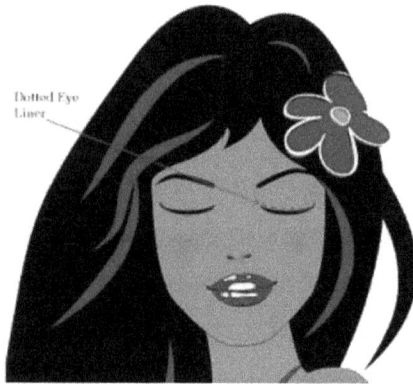

Dotted Eye Liner

4: Gaps: Ensure that there may be no hole among the attention lash and the road, if there's fill it in

5: Big Eyes: The line need to be thicker on the corners of the eyes. This will provide the illusion of large eyes

6: Double Check: Try to look for gaps and imperfections. Some eye makeup cleaner will rid of any extra or mishaps subsequently of the liquid eyeliner software program.

Mascara

Having appealing eye lashes may be the distinction among the lady next door and the lady they all dream approximately. Mascara is one of the maximum powerful makeup programs that exist and might assist make you enjoy seductive if it's miles done right.

According to principal makeup artists we are both applying mascara to the eyes wrongly or never. If you ideal mascara utility, it can be one of the most worthwhile and available make-up applications that you could ever experience.

Mascara Eyes

1) Wiggling: Pull the Mascara Brush out of the method pot and check to the lowest / roots of the lashes and wiggle the brush left and right. Wiggling should simplest be the littlest but short actions that pass left and proper

2) Carry on Wiggling: As you pass toward the suggestions preserve the brush wiggling from left to right

3) Gently comply with mascara to the lowest lash (no need to wiggle and don't positioned on too much)

Optional Steps

- You could have a take a look at with a lash comb to interrupt up the lashes (best if wished).

- To avoid Blobbing / Clumping of Mascara: Wipe Mascara Brush down with a Non-chemical tissue two times – 3 instances. This will ensure which you start with a clump unfastened brush and minimise occurrence

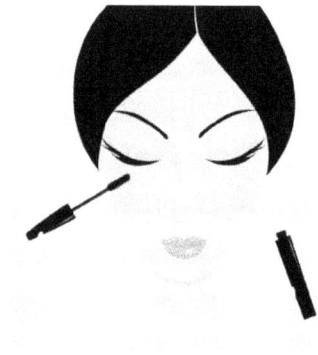

Chapter 14: Blusher

All human beings have specific face shapes and smiles. This is why you could need to apply make up blusher to a one-of-a-kind a part of your face to someone else. Good records is the techniques stay the identical.

There is considered one in all a kind advice out within the market and every make-up artists can also use a manner that fits their software program program style. The make up blusher fashion beneath is one of the most well-known and handiest to benefit, and may be tweaked to fit your dreams.

1: Smile – this may show what is typically called the 'Apple' a part of your cheeks (as hooked up thru using the photo)

2: Use a medium sized make up blush brush and dip into your preferred powder (start off with little shade) and shake off the extra

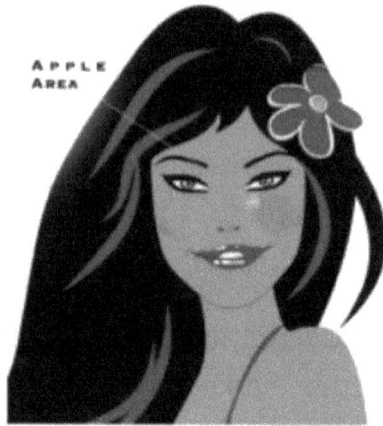

APPLE AREA

three: Starting at the lowest middle of the

'Apple', gently and softly test the color all the manner up to the temple place as demonstrated inside the Green Line photo above (the shade must fade by the point you get to the temple area, otherwise you have were given located an excessive amount of blusher on the comb or you're urgent too difficult against your pores and skin)

four: You can repeat step 3 up to 3 instances to get the arrival or definition you're after. The shape of blusher brush you use will have an effect on the overall stop of the make up software program. It is usually recommended that you put money into a expert make up blusher brush as those will assist achieve a expert appearance and could very last a long time.

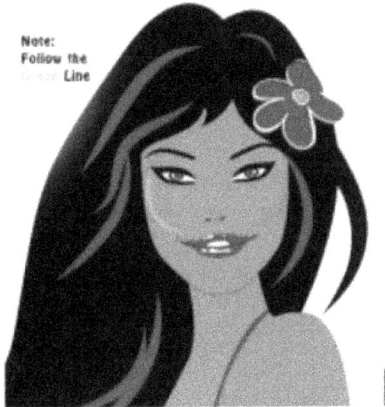

Lips

Lips add the crowning glory to any make-up software program. The lip colour have to compliment all the makeup software program software used on the facial region

Step 1

Use lip concealer along side your palms or a lip brush

Step 2:

Line the lips with a lip pencil, making sure which you keep to the natural lip line. (Lining the lips stops the lipstick bleeding onto the pores and pores and skin)

Step 3:

With the identical lip pencil fill inside the complete lip vicinity, this creates a base for the lip color and lets in the lipstick closing longer

Step 4:

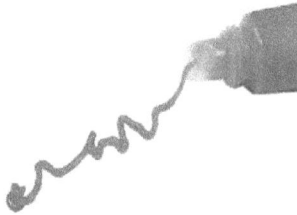

With the lip brush paint within the required lipstick to the complete lip place

Step 5:

Blot lips with tissue or upload lip gloss for extra shine

Remove Makeup

If you dispose of makeup from your face in advance than you sleep, it will assist maintain healthful pores and skin and permit your pores and skin to breath over night time. On the opposite hand if you don't take away makeup nicely you may emerge as negative your pores and pores and skin.

Needed

- Facial cleanser (buy cleaning oil in case your pores and pores and skin can be very dry)

- Eye makeup remover; and

- Quality cotton pads

Steps

1: Wash palms

2: Moisten a cotton pad with the eye makeup remover and keep positioned on your closed eye for 5 – 10 seconds before lightly wiping over the lids in an outward movement until the shadow has been removed. (Perform this step on each eyes)

3: For water resistant mascara you can need to apply a moistened cotton pad in a mild downward motion over the lashes. Repeat until mascara has been without a doubt removed

4: Cleanse the remainder of your face paying precise attention to the hair line place and the jaw line region specially if you placed on basis (cleansing techniques can also variety relying to your cleanser – whether or not or now not it's a cream based totally or foaming wash).

Use cream / oil primarily based cleanser if you commonly will be predisposed to have dry pores and skin

Do Not

- Use toddler wipes

- Scrub your face

- Over exfoliate or over cleanse

- Tug or pull your skin with the cotton pad at the same time as doing away with eye shadow

Chapter 15: The Anatomy and Physiology of the Skin

Beauty is a sensitive present.

'Beauty is a delicate gift,' stated Publius Ovidius Naso, higher known as Ovid, many centuries in the past. His smart phrases on the fragility of splendor ring real even nowadays and are in particular real of the human pores and pores and pores and skin.

The pores and pores and skin is a complex organ, the most critical in the human frame, making up about 15% of the body's weight (Kolarsick et al., 2011). You have round 19 million tiny cells in each rectangular inch of your pores and pores and skin, 1,000 nerve endings, and 20 blood vessels (Cleveland Clinic, n.D.).

So what do human organs do, and why are our organs so crucial?

Biologists define an organ as a fixed of tissues that form a shape or a unit with a specific function inside the body. The definition explains the decision of this financial disaster. The anatomy of the pores and pores and skin describes the form of the particular elements of the pores and pores and skin. Physiology describes the function of the skin and the way it works.

The pores and skin fits the definition of an organ perfectly. It includes 3 layers: the dermis, dermis, and subcutaneous fats layer. Each of these layers is uniquely constructed with unique features. If we go away aside the reality that your pores and skin is the package deal you present to the arena, the skin plays several important natural abilties:

•It protects the body from probably risky microbes and tiny residing cells. Microbes may be harmless however can also cause infections or sicknesses.

•It permits to regulate body temperature via hair coverings and sweat glands. These make sure that the human frame can tolerate temperature fluctuations with out being harmed.

•It is liable for the contact revel in. Without your pores and pores and pores and skin, you will in no way sense the softness of a infant's palms or the mildness of a spring day in your cheeks.

The pores and pores and pores and skin is sensitive but strong. It amazingly regenerates itself often and, consequently, can revel in the right sort of remedy. The fulfillment of beauty products will substantially rely on how effectively they can beautify the characteristic of the pores and pores and skin's particular layers and components.

Your pores and skin is honestly a miracle, as it's miles alive and continuously forming new cells. These cells start existence in the basal layer of the dermis and are driven to the ground, wherein they die. The miracle of the human pores and skin does no longer save you there. The useless cells, or corneocytes, are shed and changed thru new ones in a method called desquamation. Desquamation refreshes the pores and pores and pores and skin constantly as new cells come to the ground.

Knowing your pores and pores and skin will will let you make the first-rate of it and decorate your appearance and self guarantee. The better you recognise your pores and skin and its complexities, the better prepared you may be to take care of it correctly. Don't expect results right now. Your body isn't a pc in rapid-in advance mode, but you can appearance and experience better over time.

If you already regard your skin as a splendor asset, more expertise will assist you to live abreast of the maximum present day factors and generation in skincare. However, if your pores and pores and skin is the purpose of embarrassment or ache, this e book will help you understand the purpose of your pores and pores and skin trouble. Moreover, you'll get advice on addressing your pores and skin hassle with the present day-day and most advanced treatments.

The Epidermis

The epidermis can be as thin due to the fact the softest paper, but it is remarkably robust. It is thinnest for your eyelid and hundreds thicker for your arms and the soles of your toes.

The epidermis consists of severa sub-layers. Do not get forced: The pores and pores and pores and skin has 3 layers, and the dermis has 4 sub-layers. As you operate this manual, you can locate that the very outermost layer of the dermis, the stratum corneum (SC), is the point of interest of skincare.

You might in all likelihood surprise why the vain cells of the stratum corneum are so essential in pores and pores and skin care. Despite what advertisers want you to accept as real with, outside skin care products do not flow any deeper than the outer layer of the epidermis. The motive is that the cells within the uppermost layer of the pores and pores and skin are as difficult as bricks and tough to penetrate. By no manner must you give up on skin care, regardless of the fact that. The right pores and skin care merchandise interact with the moisture inside the stratum corneum and assist to seal it in.

Let us have a look at the 3 sub-layers of the epidermis. The stratum corneum, the outermost layer of the epidermis, bureaucracy the pores and pores and pores and skin barrier. The pores and pores and skin barrier is a few different time period you may again and again deal with this ebook. Just to affirm, the cells inside the stratum corneum are dead. Yes, they'll be vain, however you continue to ought to moisturise them.

The different 3 layers of the dermis – the granular, basal, and squamous – are alive. Even despite the fact that they cannot gain from topical creams, they play a vital characteristic in pores and skin exceptional.

The cells in the dermis are predominantly keratinocytes with fewer dendritic cells.

•Keratinocytes include keratin, a key component in cosmetics and hair products.

Keratin is a form of protein, and cytes is the clinical word for cells. Keratin is fibrous and the precept problem within the epidermis, hair, and nails. Keratinocytes shape a protecting layer on your pores and pores and pores and skin, and collectively they make up the backbone of your epidermis.

•Dendritic cells are critical in the pores and skin's immune responses. They are also located within the lining of the nose, lungs, belly, and intestines.

00001.Jpeg

Regeneration of the Epidermis

Remember, the epidermis has its non-public sub-layers. These layers are dynamic and undergo normal regeneration. In more youthful human beings, it takes the cells round 28 days to transport from the basal layer to the topmost useless layer (stratum corneum) (Kolarsick et al., 2011). This manner slows down with age, even though.

Skin regeneration in ladies 50 and older might take in to 80 4 days, relying on food plan, pores and pores and skin care routine, hydration degrees, and environmental elements (Walters, 2022).

Keep this timespan in thoughts even as you squeeze a pimple. Squeezing damages the delicate cells on your epidermis, and the opportunities are accurate that the encircling place also can get inflamed. Even in case you get the pus out, it leaves a purple, inflamed, and ugly wound. Healing is based upon on new cellular formation. It technique you have to wait anyways for the broken cells to be shed and the new ones emigrate to the surface. Instead of forcing the zit to pop, you dispose of the recovery.

As the trendy cells circulate from the basal layer, they form attachment plates that interact and connect to one-of-a-type plates. These connections toughen the pores and pores and skin and help form the shape and form of your face.

As the cells migrate upward, they lose moisture and eventually die. At this level, they end up hard and are called corneocytes. Corneocytes might be dead, however they will absorb small portions of moisture that keep your pores and pores and skin hydrated.

Scientists and splendor researchers are continuously mastering and growing merchandise based totally on the dermis's capability to renew itself via transferring vintage cells to the floor. Through the centuries, and specially over the past a long time, beauty research has benefitted immensely from medical studies, specifically concerning wound recuperation.

The Basal Layer on the Bottom of the Epidermis

New cellular formation takes place in the basal layer at the lowest of the epidermis. Cell regeneration within the basal layer starts at the same time as the keratinocytes (the cells containing the protein keratin) divide rapidly.

New cells are driven upward to make space for even greater moderen cells.

Distributed some of the keratinocytes are melanocytes, cells with very particular capabilities. In a complex approach (given right here in a simplified version), melanocytes produce melanin, a pigment that includes amino acids.

The colour of your pores and pores and skin is predicated upon in large part on the amount of melanin produced thru the melanocytes. The amount of melanin in your pores and skin additionally determines whether or no longer you tan brown or clearly flip crimson. It even determines whether or now not you'll increase freckles. Remember, your pores and pores and pores and skin color is likewise inspired via the amount of time you spend within the sun, your hormones, and your genes.

The melanocytes produce melanin in the basal layer. The melanin then moves into the keratinocytes. Melanin's primary function is to defend you from the dangerous impact of ultraviolet radiation.

The Squamous Layer of the Epidermis

The squamous layer is proper above the basal layer and is the thickest part of the dermis. As the name suggests, the cells on this layer appear like fish scales. The cells in the squamous layer moreover connect with different cells to shape a protecting barrier in competition to accidents and bodily stress.

The Granular Layer of the Epidermis

The granular layer is the top residing layer of the epidermis. The granular layer at the fingers and feet is understandably thicker than at the face.

The cells inside the granular layer consist typically of gentle keratin in assessment to the hard keratin in hair and nails. As the mobile moves thru the granular layer, it loses moisture, will become more difficult, and sooner or later ultimately finally ends up dry and useless within the stratum corneum.

The Stratum Corneum

We are really decrease back at the topmost layer, the stratum corneum, with lifeless cells. As stated in advance, maximum splendor products don't flow deeper than the stratum corneum. If these cells are vain, does it make any experience to feed them with pricey moisturisers? Would petroleum jelly now not protect the pores and pores and skin as successfully from dehydration?

The answer is plain: Yes. You need to moisturise your skin diligently. Modern moisturisers and serums are scientifically formulated to prevent dehydration. Also, many current-day products contain humectants, an agent that retains moisture inside the useless cells of the stratum corneum. And yes, petroleum jelly is useful to hold the pores and pores and pores and skin's herbal moisture intact.

The cornified cells in the stratum corneum are critical to shield the pores and pores and skin, as they maintain moisture and save you risky substances from penetrating the pores and pores and skin. Furthermore, the ones cells are programmed to die, a gadget called programmed loss of existence. Programmed loss of life illustrates how tough and specific the human pores and pores and pores and skin is.

Usually, vain tissue affects the neighbouring tissue as well, however in programmed death, the mobile dies without any harm to the surrounding cells. On pinnacle of that, due to the truth the mobile dies, a cutting-edge one takes its area. Skincare merchandise goal the more moderen cells, as they will absorb moisture and plumb out and make your pores and pores and skin appearance more energizing.

Theoretically, harmful microbes can enter the pores and skin through the tiny openings a number of the vain corneocytes and moreover through the openings of the hair follicles. But the frame has an remarkable defence system. Lipids (the oils in the pores and skin) accumulate within the ones mini-openings a few of the corneocytes, and sebum fills the hair follicles. Together they shape a natural barrier to maintain volatile molecules and dirt out.

Unfortunately, this barrier additionally prevents beauty elements from getting into the granular, squamous, or basal layers of the epidermis. In a outstanding worldwide, one might also have wanted for the skin care products to penetrate the pores and pores and pores and skin deeply, even reaching the dermis in which collagen is long-established. Unfortunately, pores and skin care lotions do no longer even get to the basal layer to shape new cells.

Several splendor houses these days claimed that newly superior merchandise include peptides and that their products stimulate collagen production. It is exciting records, but regrettably, clinical findings need to be supported thru massive-scale research and peer-evaluated publications in clinical journals. Up till now, not sufficient scientific proof is available. Nonetheless, the opportunity that peptides need to stimulate the producing of collagen and elastin is typically welcomed. It is said in extra element inside the bankruptcy on pores and skin merchandise and key substances.

It is crucial to differentiate among splendor products and scientific remedies along side nicotine and hormonal patches. These patches do in the end acquire the bloodstream and feature lengthy-time period outcomes. Cosmetic products, even though, have first-rate a quick-time period localised effect at the pores and skin.

Cosmeceutical research is a fairly new subject that mixes physics, chemistry, and biology inside the quest for cosmetics that still have a therapeutic effect on the pores and skin. As studies maintains, we are able to count on thrilling new merchandise and technology.

Epidermal Appendages

Hair, nails, and the numerous sweat glands form a part of the human pores and pores and skin's epidermal appendages. They are interesting skills, as they expand from the outside inward. The system starts offevolved already at some stage in the embryo level inside the womb.

A female's hair is known as her final touch, and properly-stored nails ooze sophistication, but hair and nails are plenty more than just aesthetic functions. They carry out important capabilities in the body.

Sweat Glands

Sweat glands is probably lots tons less glamorous, but they are although important in our our bodies. Humans have 3 various kinds of sweat glands, and those at the face are referred to as eccrine sweat glands. We typically accomplice sweat with an unpleasant odour, but the eccrine (facial) sweat glands' secretion is odourless.

(Do now not confuse the eccrine glands with the apocrine glands inside the armpits. The latter glands are the smelly culprits, as they secrete a thick fluid that, even as it comes into touch with the skin's surface, reasons an unsightly odour.)

The smooth sweat produced through the facial eccrine glands is right for the pores and skin in more than one way. It allows to cool the frame, specially eventually of exercise and on heat days. Evaporation motives cooling, and the body cools down even as the sweat evaporates.

Sweat has a few exciting additional benefits on your pores and skin. It has immoderate water content material material material and as a result hydrates the pores and pores and skin. It additionally consists of urea and uric acid, suitable moisturisers for dry pores and skin.

Furthermore, the minerals and salt in the sweat characteristic an exfoliate, and that they truely clean the pores and skin. They wash micro organism, dirt debris, and impurities from the pores. It rids the skin of pollution, and the immune device is automatically boosted.

If you're nonetheless no longer happy that sweat may be actual in your pores and skin, check your pores and pores and skin after a strenuous workout session. You can be sparkling; your pores and skin will appearance hydrated and more energizing.

Hair Follicles

Did you normally need thicker hair and attempted many products that promised you honestly that? Here is the awful news. You are born with a specific extensive form of hair follicles that appear in a one-of-a-type sample over your head and body. It is a given, and now not anything you may do can trade your hair kind or the capability amount of hair for your head. (However, if you want to dispose of greater hair, Chapter 7 tells you the whole thing approximately electrolysis and why you should not be fearful of it.)

The tiny hair follicle is a miracle in itself. It might be small, but it's far intricately built with numerous additives. The sebaceous gland develops as a tiny bud at the bottom of the follicle, but greater at the sebaceous gland later.

Small Muscle Bundle

Below the sebaceous gland is a small and easy muscle bundle deal connected to the follicle's root sheath. The tiny muscle bundles comprise stem cells that have the potential to regenerate the hair follicle. Thus, in case you pluck out the hair with the follicle, the muscle package deal deal remains within the again of and, consequently, a cutting-edge follicle will regrow. It may want to probable make the effort, but in the long run, your hair follicle may be regenerated and new hair will expand due to each unique tiny miracle at the bottom of the hair follicle, the hair bulb.

Hair Bulb

The hair bulb holds even extra surprises. While the muscle package deal deal is responsible for the regrowth of the hair follicle, the bulb is liable for the growth of the hair shaft. The hair bulb's matrix cells proliferate suddenly, producing the hair shaft, its inner root sheath, and its outer root sheath.

That long, clean hair you're so glad with (or choice so intensely) stems from the tiny bulbs at the lowest of the hair follicles. The form and size of the inner root sheath decide the shape of your hair texture – without delay, wavy, or curly.

Hair grows in 3 ranges. During the number one anagen phase, the hair grows actively. The increase section can final among 3 to 5 years. After the increase diploma follows the catagen segment, while the follicle shrinks. The hair separates from the follicle but remains in area. During the last section, or telogen segment, the hair follicle takes a rest for a couple of months (WebMD, 2010).

Getting gray hair is a part of growing older, and the muse of your grey hair lies within the hair bulb. It's time for a bit of simplified technological data another time: The hair bulb includes melanocytes, the same cells as within the basal layer. As the call indicates, melanocytes incorporate melanin, contributing to pores and pores and skin and hair colour. However, with age, the melanocytes produce a lot less and masses much less melanin, and the hair will become step by step lighter. Consequently, because the melanocytes age, you become with grey hair.

Fortunately, contemporary hair dyes can solve the hassle. Alternatively, you may enjoy the softness that your particular coloration of gray brings to your abilties. Once the greying has began out, the method cannot be became spherical, and you'll in no way regain your precise hair coloration.

Redheads are particular, as they have got a genetic model that produces greater pink melanin to make a redhead stand out most of the relaxation of the population. Redheads, have amusing your location of information!

Nails

Your nails had been now not speculated to be decorations however are there to defend the arms and feet. Nonetheless, polished and neat nails do spherical off a properly-stored appearance. The opposite is likewise real; your nails are a positive giveaway if you don't take care of your self.

Nails consist within the predominant of keratin, and, as we apprehend, keratin strengthens your pores and pores and pores and skin, hair, and nails. The visible part of your nail is lifeless, much like the hair shaft and the stratum corneum, the outermost layer of your pores and pores and pores and skin. Therefore, you can lessen your nails without any ache. However, you have some feeling within the nails because of the nerve endings inside the epidermis right now under the nail.

Also, beneath the nail bed, you have got were given tiny capillaries that feed the nail bed. Nails develop quicker in summer time than in the wintry weather. Interestingly, the nails on your dominant hand develop faster than the nails however. Scientists recollect that prolonged blood flow to the dominant hand stimulates nail growth.

Look out:

•Be privy to coloration modifications in the nails, as a change in colour may advocate an underlying health hassle which encompass fungi, thyroid illness, diabetes, or psoriasis.

•Your grandmother grow to be incorrect while she stated calcium shortage brought about her white spots. The white is because of accidents, by way of and huge so small that you don't even phrase it.

•Many ladies are involved approximately the horizontal traces on their nails. They are the stop give up result of pressure and, even though harmless, are a warning that you need to address your self for a exchange. Also, no matter the reality that nail-biting is harmless, it is unhygienic and need to be avoided.

•Well-saved nails do not have to be painted. Unpolished nails can no matter the fact that be nicely-stored, easy, and attractive. Moreover, your nails have to get sufficient breathing time. Nail polish and varnish removers damage the nails at the same time as used constantly. Thus, deliver your nails a chance to recover.

•Handle your cuticles with care. They defend the nail base; consequently, don't lessen away too harshly.

Sebaceous Glands

The sebaceous glands are the closing but now not the least of the appendages of the epidermis to speak about. As you may see from the names, those glands produce sebum, a natural lipid moisturising pores and pores and skin. The sebocytes produce sebum and, like keratinocytes, sebocytes are also programmed to die. As the sebocytes dissolve, they release sebum into the hair follicle.

The sebum is pushed to the floor as herbal lubrication for the pores and skin and the scalp. But if an excessive amount of sebum is released, you may boom a pores and pores and skin trouble.

The sebaceous glands are important in all sorts of zits and can cause havoc at the pores and pores and skin. Chapter 6 discusses those glands and their feature in acne in element.

Dermo-Epidermal Junction

The dermis and the dermis meet at the dermo-epidermal junction. It is a multi-layered membrane that holds the dermis and the epidermis together. It supports the dermis and plays a number one characteristic in getting oxygen, vitamins, and fluids to the dermis. The membrane is porous, which lets in movement for nourishment upward and waste depend downward.

Additionally, the dermo-epidermal membrane strengthens the skin and offers safety in opposition to accidents from the outdoor.

The Dermis

The epidermis is the most critical issue of the pores and skin and similarly allows the epidermis. It bureaucracy a cushion for the dermis to rest on, consequently shielding the touchy epidermis.

Although beauty products do not penetrate the dermis, a wholesome dermis is critical for pores and skin health. It feeds the epidermis and protects it. It contributes to the skin's pliability and elasticity, binds water, regulates temperature, and lets in to your touch sense.

The epidermis includes a community of connective tissue and blood vessels. The dermis does no longer have any blood vessels, so it relies upon on the epidermis for nourishment and waste elimination.

The dermis and the dermis (except for the outermost stratum corneum) are living components of your pores and pores and skin. They interact with every wonderful thru the dermo-epidermal junction. The epidermal appendages (hair, nails, sweat, and sebaceous glands mentioned above) are a part of the cooperation and interaction amongst the ones layers of the skin.

The dermis is specifically interesting because it's far composed in particular of collagen, elastin, and hyaluronic acid, buzzwords in modern-day-day pores and skin care.

Natural Substances within the Dermis

Collagen

Collagen is the essential protein inside the dermis and paperwork about 70% of the dermis (Kolarsick, 2011). Collagen isn't always completely positioned inside the dermis. The tendons, ligaments, and bone linings additionally have this form of protein. It confirms how important collagen is, in and for the human frame.

Collagen gives strength and provides resilience to the pores and skin, as it includes protein fibres that shape a connective network referred to as fibroblasts. The network (together with different pores and pores and skin components) is responsible for the architectural framework of the frame (Alberts, 2002). Think of the fibroblasts giving form to your pores and pores and skin as your teeth offer shape to your mouth.

Fibroblasts play a extensive characteristic in wound healing. When the pores and pores and skin is injured, the fibroblasts across the area proliferate and convey massive numbers of unique cells that sell recuperation and spoil down the fibrin clot.

Like many unique cells in human pores and pores and skin, collagen cells are not static but are continuously converting. In layperson's phrases, they get vintage and crumble, but new cells form continuously. The pores and pores and pores and skin is certainly a living and dynamic organ, an extremely good reason a excellent manner to look after it. Collagen in pores and pores and skin products and collagen nutritional supplements are said inside the following two chapters.

Elastin

Elastin is made from numerous protein molecules and, proper to its call, elastin can stretch and reduce lower again. It is why your pores and skin returns to its shape at the same time as it is stretched or pinched.

Unfortunately, with age, the pores and pores and skin's elasticity reduces as heaps much less elastin is produced. Too an lousy lot solar publicity reasons ultraviolet radiation that destroys elastin manufacturing, a way called photoaging. If you care for your skin, it's far crucial to save you sun harm in any respect charges. You can not forestall the natural developing old system, but you can do masses to prevent solar harm. You can take a look at greater about photoaging and hyperpigmentation in Chapter five and Chapter nine.

Hyaluronic Acid

Hyaluronic acid isn't a protein but a herbal water-binding substance within the epidermis, additionally decided in the eyes. Although now not as considerable as collagen or elastin, hyaluronic acid is important for preserving moisture within the pores and skin.

It controls tissue hydration thru preserving massive quantities of water. Hyaluronic acid is a herbal lubricator in moderate tissue.

Medical specialists use hyaluronic acid in wound recuperation, and splendor technology has benefitted drastically from medical research on this discipline. It has anti-inflammatory and antibacterial houses. When the pores and pores and skin is injured, the encircling cells increase the production of hyaluronic acid to help within the restoration technique.

More Structures within the Dermis

Blood vessels

The dermis has a network of blood vessels. The blood vessels in the uppermost layer of the epidermis are tiny capillaries. The blood vessels deeper inside the epidermis and the epidermis-subcutaneous junction are more massive and are furnished with sparkling blood thru large blood vessels.

It is essential to keep in thoughts that the dermis does now not have any blood vessels. The dermis relies upon at the small capillaries inside the top a part of the epidermis for a supply of oxygen, nourishment, and fluids. These small capillaries moreover take away the waste from the dermis. Following the rule of nature, oxygen and nutrients circulate from the better interest inside the capillaries to the 'empty' cells in the dermis. In the identical way, the waste is channelled thru the capillaries to the blood vessels and the kidneys.

The network of superficial and deeper blood vessels within the dermis is crucial in regulating the body's temperature. The pores and pores and skin does no longer adjust the temperature in isolation, in spite of the truth that. It works with the hypothalamus placed within the thoughts, every distinctive example of approaches wonderfully hard the human body is.

The hypothalamus attempts to hold your frame temperature at around 37°C. When the body receives too heat, the hypothalamus instructs the capillaries inside the dermis to widen. More blood actions into the capillaries and warmth is launched into the air; therefore, the frame cools down. When the body receives too bloodless, the hypothalamus sends the possibility message. The capillaries constrict, the blood go with the flow will increase, and warmth is contained.

If you have got were given ever wondered wherein warmth flushes originate, contemporary research hyperlinks menopausal warm flushes to modifications inside the capillaries (Hazell, 2011).

Muscles inside the Dermis

The facial muscle mass are controlled thru a cranial nerve that splits into numerous smaller nerves, which then go to unique facial regions. These nerves permit humans to particular various emotions and feelings. And at the identical time as you don't want to show your proper emotions, you may cleverly manipulate the ones nerves to cowl your actual mind.

You also can surprise why data on facial functions is covered in a skin care manual. Have you ever seen a stunning grumpy woman? How you enjoy and the way you view the arena indicates in your face. When you smile from your soul, you are lots more appealing than a forced or faux smile. Your facial expressions reveal your feelings and intellectual u . S . A .. However, in unguarded moments, your face could likely deliver away what you need to cover.

Facial expressions are quite a top notch deal an global language. A smile is a grin, whether or not you're excellent in Samoa or Saudi. A frown is a frown, no matter your foul temper in France or Finland. Smiling and frowning are only of the infinite messages we supply others without talking a word. Furthermore, you can smile with surely one nook of the mouth, or huge and with an open mouth and eyes. It is the motive why data on what number of muscle mass you use for smiling range lots.

Your facial muscle organizations originate from the skull and protrude into the dermis. They art work collectively to bring movement for your cheeks, eyebrows, eyelids, forehead, upper and decrease lips, nose, and nostrils. And in case you are wonderful, even your ears! Only among 10 and 20% of the population can wiggle their ears (Joi, 2009).

Your facial muscular tissues aren't quality concerned in expression but additionally assist in identifying non-public look. They defend the eyes and play a function in speaking, creating a track, and consuming – they even prevent drooling.

Mast Cells

Mast cells are the epidermis's resident anti-inflammatory combatants. They help within the fight in the direction of zits, and you may studies extra approximately mast cells inside the financial disaster on acne. They release histamine to counteract hypersensitive reactions and kick in proper away after an harm. Mast cells additionally stimulate the growth of keratinocytes.

The Hypodermis, or Subcutaneous Fat Layer

Right at the bottom of the pores and pores and skin is a fatty layer called the hypodermis. There are few things women like less than fats. Fat is appeared due to the fact the baddie, and we frequently want it away. However, the hypodermis gives the number one structural resource for the pores and pores and skin. It connects the pores and pores and skin with the bones and muscle groups, providing you with specific facial functions.

The fats layer offers form on your face; without it, you may have a ghostly and sunken look. Without the fat layer, human beings might in all likelihood appearance downright scary.

Furthermore, it protects in competition to injuries, promotes pores and pores and skin restore, and regulates hair regeneration tempo. It insulates the frame from temperature fluctuations. But this fatty layer has one more surprise: It produces leptin, the hormone that tells the frame it has had sufficient to devour! How are we able to not love fatty hypodermis? It is crucial for our seems and nudges us to consume much less!

Quick Reminder

cytes: generally used as a suffix, because of this that mobile corneocytes: the lifeless cells on the outermost layer of the pores and pores and skin, consisting on the entire of keratin

fibroblasts: cells inside the connective tissue of the pores and pores and skin that deliver shape and convey collagen

keratinocytes: a cell that produces keratin

dendritic: an immune mobile

melanocytes: a cell that produces melanin, the colour pigment

matrix cell: a mobile that would trade from fluid to a gel and reduce once more to fluid

mast cellular: a cell that releases histamine to fight infection

General Terminology

anatomy: how the pores and skin is installed

appendages: down growth from the pores and skin inward for the duration of the embryo diploma (hair, nails, sure glands, and many others.)

cranial nerve: a set of paired nerves at the back of the thoughts that sends electric powered messages

desquamation: a herbal tool wherein the dead cells on the pores and skin are shed to make vicinity for logo spanking new cells

programmed demise: herbal loss of existence of a mobile to make way for a new mobile

frame shape: the pores and skin's function

squamous: looks like fish scales

glands: an organ that makes materials

apocrine glands: sweat glands inside the armpits

eccrine glands: sweat glands at the face

sebaceous gland: a gland that produces sebum inside the hair follicle

Substances

collagen: most vital protein positioned in the skin

elastin: protein discovered inside the pores and skin, helps pores and pores and skin to stretch and go returned to its authentic form and duration

hyaluronic acid: water-binding molecules with an vital characteristic in severa physiological strategies that help with collagen and elastin production

lipids: oils in the skin

fatty acids: a form of lipid

urea: waste product generated through using the breakdown of proteins

uric acid: a waste product determined inside the blood

Chapter 16: Skin Type and Identification

Everything has splendor, but now not anybody sees it.

Sadly, Confucius modified into proper. Many women don't see their private splendor. From early early life, we're conditioned to evaluate ourselves to the right photos of celebrities within the media. We neglect that the ones ladies have make-up teams, hairdressers, and probable private shoppers who paintings as a manufacturing employer to offer a expert 'product' to the arena.

Moreover, the virtual digicam team makes use of every to be had technological tool to create an suave surrender product. Ten to 1, celebrities appearance extensively lots much less extremely good when they awaken in the morning to the desires of a difficult day.

During the past a few years, social media has grow to be a effective pressure and plays a significant feature in our social and private lives. Of path, social media is in no way best poor. On the contrary, it has severa advantages: It connects us to the area, broadens our horizons, and enriches our private lives. We assemble stimulating relationships, percent every others' evaluations, and benefit know-how via the internet.

Since the start of time, look has been important, and it even though is. Visual conversation has constantly been a part of lifestyles; many examples exist in animal lifestyles. Male birds use their colourful feathers to draw ladies. Chimpanzees decorate their palms and slap the floor to intimidate. The poison dart frog is colourful orange, caution predators now not to eat them (Khan Academy, n.D.).

Similarly, over the centuries, humans have used visual communique consciously or subconsciously to show recognition and splendor and ship non-verbal messages. Generally, handsome humans are rated greater a achievement and famous than their plainer colleagues.

Social media has taken visible verbal exchange to a great degree, with overemphasis at the outward appearance and no longer reflecting any of the internal trends of the character. Most social media clients publish selfies portraying themselves in the high-quality mild possible. Furthermore, we're constantly confronted via pix of stunning humans on our displays.

We recognize that with telephone technology, those snap shots are photoshopped into close to-ideal pix. Still, one's conceitedness might also go through even as comparing oneself with remarkable photographs.

In a cutting-edge-day article published within the European Scientific Journal, researchers cautioned that 88% of Facebook users compared themselves with online pictures. Moreover, the researchers discovered a strong indication that self-esteem reduced with the boom in time spent on Facebook (Jan, 2017).

Back to Confucius' terms. You are specific. You need to discover ways to recognize and internalise it. You might not have the shape of hair that developments in the interim. You might be overweight or have awful pores and skin. But somewhere there lurks a well-saved and cared-for model of you. Perhaps a go to to an excellent hairdresser, a dermatologist, and ordinary walks with the canine are desired to reveal the better-looking you.

Take examine: Beauty has awesome dimensions. Of path, hair, pores and pores and skin, and being properly-built make contributions to your splendor. But being properly-cared for and properly-saved are critical elements of being attractive, if no longer stunning, in traditional terms. It is proper for every age but turns into increasingly more essential as a woman a long term. A well-saved woman is an appealing girl.

Here's the trap 22 situation, although: Sometimes existence breaks your vanity down little by little, and also you get caught in the youngsters' programmes, your companion's lives, and your troubles. Your unconscious tells you that your circle of relatives want to return first. In the device, you start neglecting your self.

Admittedly, it's far difficult to enjoy stunning if you speed thru the days like a bullet educate thru the Russian steppes. Maybe that is the time for a cliché: You must appreciate yourself and your unique appears to regain arrogance.

Of path, there will continually be a extra attractive individual than you. Still, deep down, you need to go through in thoughts that your look does no longer determine your price as a person or ladies. Besides, the ones pix you jealously admire are not even true.

Recent studies opinions that self-care and properly-being are more and more seemed as fitness problems. A wholesome manner of life is crucial for a healthful body. A healthy frame, over again, is a prerequisite for accurate pores and skin. Appearance has as a stop result come to be a health problem, and self-care is important to look nicely and be healthful. Fitness, healthy consuming, and private body and skincare are commonly trendy due to the reality the norm in current society.

Join this fitness-is-splendor style these days. You can't experience cute if you aren't healthful and properly-stored. Does this sound a chunk like pie inside the sky? Let us then get all of the manner down to the fundamentals. Start loving yourself with a few minutes right here and there. As one of the large names in pores and skin care and cosmetics says so regularly in their advertising flashes: 'Because you're nicely worth it.'

Your skin is the triumphing wrapping; you are the actual gift. You gift yourself to the location wrapped beautifully or carelessly for your pores and pores and pores and skin. Your pores and pores and pores and skin is often the primary element others see and select you on. Your pores and pores and skin tells the tale of methods you deal with your self earlier than you even communicate a word.

Look at yourself within the rest room mirror. Are you glad with what you be aware? You want your particular present wrapping to be of the super brilliant and to appearance as actual as feasible for yourself.

There are specific strategies to classify pores and pores and skin sorts, which are not typically in opposition. On the other, the splendor industry is privileged to apply clinical studies to supply pores and pores and skin care based on sound research and clinical expertise. We will discuss the 2 systems in the fundamental used, the first a medical and the second a cosmetic beauty of pores and skin. Several structures had been superior thru the severa years, and your clinical practitioner may also moreover use a unique one.

The Medical Way – Fitzpatrick Skin Type (FST)

Since 1975, dermatologists and cosmetologists have used the Fitzpatrick Skin Type (FST) device to classify pores and skin types primarily based mostly on their reaction to the sun. It should be confused that this device does not classify pores and skin sorts in keeping with ethnic organizations. The category grow to be in no manner based totally mostly on skin shade or ethnic enterprise however on how the pores and skin reacts to sunburn.

Since 1975 scientific doctors have used FST to decide how patients' pores and pores and skin reacts to sunburn. It end up completed via self-assessment interviews. The consequences received on this method were semi-subjective, as people had specific interpretations of the terminology used within the questionnaires. Scientists and scientific clinical docs agree that best dermatologists or clinical practitioners want to do FST kind.

Your pores and pores and skin's response to ultraviolet rays of the sun relies upon on the melanin degrees inside the keratinocytes. Melanin protects the pores and skin towards ultraviolet rays.

Because self-evaluation is not accurate, some dermatologists use a complex clinical approach to diploma the melanin in the pores and skin. Reflectance spectrophotometry determines the pores and pores and skin's response to the solar based totally totally on pores and pores and pores and skin reflectance. Unfortunately, those exams are not yet commonly available.

Fitzpatrick Skin Type I to VI

Based at the Fitzpatrick technique, six pores and pores and pores and skin kinds were recognized, each with precise tendencies. Please take a look at that you can no longer in shape precisely into one kind quality but is probably a mixture of two types.

Skin maximum cancers is crucial; if dubious, are looking for recommendation from a professional if you have some thing bothering you. Knowing your FST is essential to information your threat of pores and pores and skin most cancers and shielding your self hence.

Skin Type 1

•The herbal skin colour is relatively sincere.

•The natural hair coloration is mild blond or pink.

•The eye coloration is blue, slight gray, or moderate inexperienced.

•When uncovered to the solar, the pores and skin burns freckles.

•It continually burns and in no manner tans.

Skin Type 2

•The herbal skin coloration is sincere.

•The herbal hair shade is blond.

•The eye color is blue, grey, or inexperienced.

•When exposed to the solar, the pores and pores and skin usually has freckles, burns, and peels.

•It not often tans.

Skin Types 1 and a couple of: What to Know and What to Do

•You receives solar damage from exposure.

•The sun will age your pores and skin.

•You have a immoderate danger of growing cancer or skin most cancers.

•Use sunscreen with a excessive sun protection difficulty (SFP), a hat, and solar shades that block ultraviolet rays.

•Stay out of the sun and within the coloration as a good buy as possible and put on protecting apparel.

•Check yourself for modifications to your pores and skin each month and visit your medical medical medical doctor as quickly as a yr for a radical check-up.

Skin Type 3

•The natural pores and skin colour is trustworthy to beige.

•The natural hair shade is darkish blond to moderate brown.

•The eye shade is hazel to moderate brown.

•When exposed to the solar, the pores and pores and pores and skin once in a while freckles.

•The pores and skin every so often burns and on occasion tans.

Skin Type 4

•The herbal pores and skin color is mild brown and frequently defined as olive.

•The natural hair coloration is dark brown.

•The eye shade is dark brown.

•When uncovered to the solar, the pores and pores and skin commonly does not freckle or burn.

•The skin tans well.

Skin Type five

•The herbal pores and skin coloration is darkish brown.

•The herbal hair colour is darkish brown to black.

•The eye shade is dark brown to black.

•When exposed to the sun, the pores and skin not regularly develops freckles and does not burn.

•The pores and pores and skin typically tans.

Skin Type 6

•The herbal pores and skin shade is dark brown.

•The herbal hair coloration is black.

•The eye shade is brown-black.

•When exposed to the sun, the pores and pores and skin in no manner has freckles and in no way burns.

•The pores and pores and skin tans darkly.

Skin Types 3, 4, 5, and 6: What to Know and What to Do

•You are though at risk of sun damage and signs and symptoms and symptoms of having antique.

•You are vulnerable to skin maximum cancers, in particular if you have used a sunbed for tanning or have had not unusual publicity to the sun.

•Many sufferers with darker skin put off going to their doctor, as they falsely remember darker pores and pores and skin isn't at risk of pores and pores and skin most cancers. An early prognosis of most cancers can keep your life.

•Use sunscreen with a sun protection component (SFP) of as a minimum 15, a hat, and sunglasses that block ultraviolet rays.

•Stay out of the solar and in the colour as a good deal as feasible.

•Wear protecting apparel in case you are within the solar for lengthy intervals.

•Check your whole body for changes for your pores and skin every month.

•Visit your doctor as soon as a year for an extensive test-up. People with darker pores and skin can also get Acral lentiginous most cancers. This shape of pores and pores and pores and skin maximum cancers appears on a part of the frame that have come to be no longer uncovered to the solar. Therefore, those melanomas are regularly high-quality determined at a past due diploma whilst they are hard to address efficaciously (Hecht, 2019).

The Cosmetic Way – Skin Condition and Needs

Cosmetic scientists approach pores and skin care from a extraordinary component of view than clinical researchers. Cosmetic generation desires to beautify your appears at the identical time as the scientific profession addresses fitness troubles. However, a dermatologist is also expert that will help you with conditions which includes hyperpigmentation, acne, and different situations. These won't be life-threatening but may additionally have destructive physical and emotional results. Together, beauty and clinical sciences let you take care of your pores and skin and maintain precise pores and skin first-rate.

The beauty corporation has contributed notably to the overall public's converting opinion on the want of safety closer to UV radiation and pores and skin cancer. Although skin care merchandise are designed to preserve moisture, cosmeceutical experts moreover emphasise safety in opposition to the solar – a double whammy for the skin. Be warned, despite the fact that, that you can't rely upon pores and skin care merchandise to protect the pores and pores and skin in the direction of the sun; sunscreen is a need.

Cosmetic products motive to maintain the pores and pores and pores and skin well-balanced and healthy; no longer too dry, no longer too oily. Moisture is an essential locating out element in pores and skin type, and beauty scientists classify the skin constant with its moisture degree, sebaceous secretion, and sensitivity (Almarill, n.D.).

Every pores and pores and skin is incredible, and excellent if you have determined your pores and skin type can you're making informed options on skincare products and remedies.

The beauty industry has diagnosed five pores and pores and skin sorts, and research specializes inside the character wishes of the 5 pores and skin sorts.

Cosmetic Industry Skin Types

Normal Skin

Normal pores and pores and skin is a few factor however normal; it is the nice pores and skin kind, however few ladies have everyday skin. Normal pores and pores and skin is neither dry nor oily. It has a honest texture, with out a obvious pores or discolouring. The pores and pores and skin appears clean and moderate – each woman's dream, however sadly, no longer the reality for optimum girls. Most women battle with a few factor of their skin.

Sensitive Skin

Sensitive pores and pores and pores and skin is sensitive and reacts to environmental stimuli which incorporates the solar, warm temperature, and bloodless climate. The pores and pores and skin barrier is not robust enough to guard the pores and pores and skin; consequently, the pores and skin is with out issues angry. This form of pores and pores and skin frequently has rashes, infections, or hypersensitive reactions.

Some talk with this pores and skin type as indignant pores and pores and skin. It is noticeably dry, feels tight, and is crimson and itchy.

Dry Skin

Dry pores and skin stocks a number of the signs of sensitive pores and pores and pores and skin. Dry pores and skin might be genetic, however it could also be attributed to hormonal modifications.

Often, outside elements dehydrate the pores and skin. Air conditioners, hot water, the sun, tanning beds, and lengthy, heat baths or showers reason dehydration. Avoid immoderate bloodless, warmness, and air conditioners as a top notch deal as feasible. Harsh elements in cleaners, especially soaps and pores and skin care merchandise, additionally get worse dryness. If your pores and pores and skin is dry notwithstanding regular moisturising, change your cleaner to a non-foaming one. You is probably aware a proper away development.

Certain medicinal capsules moreover purpose dry pores and pores and skin, and you need to speak it together with your clinical doctor or pharmacist.

Dry pores and pores and pores and skin seems stupid and dehydrated with traces however has no visible pores. However, the pores and pores and skin is much less elastic and shows early signs of growing older. Regular moisturising will skip far to hydrate your pores and pores and pores and skin.

Oily Skin

Oily pores and skin generally has enlarged pores and a barely greasy floor. Oily pores and skin is frequently genetic. The sebaceous glands produce greater sebum, a fats that motives a glittery complexion.

People more youthful than 30 frequently be afflicted by oily pores and skin due to the fact hormonal imbalances stimulate greater sebum manufacturing.

Combination Skin

Combination pores and skin typically has dry and oily regions. The so-known as T-zone (forehead, nostril and chin) has greater sebaceous glands which produce an excessive amount of sebum. These areas appear great with blackheads and visible pores. The skin on the cheeks is ordinary or dry.

Baumann Skin Type Indicator (BSTI)

Professor Leslie Baumann, a specially real researcher, published drastically on pores and skin types, and lots of beauty companies base their digital assessment fashions on Baumann's studies. She is a splendor dermatologist and advanced a questionnaire to decide pores and skin kind on the University of Miami in 2004. This questionnaire remains substantially utilized by researchers, beauty homes, medical professionals, beauticians, and people.

It is critical to keep in mind that Baumann's machine is based totally totally on individual pores and skin houses; Fitzpatrick's gadget is based totally virtually on the pores and pores and skin's response to the sun and the chance of pores and skin most cancers. The structures do now not oppose each unique. You have to be acquainted with every. Baumann's category will permit you to pick out the right pores and skin care products. Fitzpatrick's class will assist guard your pores and skin within the course of solar damage and the opportunity of pores and pores and skin most cancers.

Leslie Baumann designed a digital-based totally questionnaire to evaluate 4 essential houses of the pores and skin: oily as opposed to dry, sensitive in preference to resistant, pigmented in preference to non-pigmented, and wrinkled as opposed to unwrinkled. These four pores and skin types are further defined in terms of the skin's residences or obstacles to pores and skin health: dehydration, infection, pigmentation, and growing vintage (Baumann, 2008).

www.ingramcontent.com/pod-product-compliance
Lightning Source LLC
Chambersburg PA
CBHW060223030426
42335CB00014B/1323